Soft Tissue Therapy for the Lower Limb

Hands-On Guides for Therapists

T0293418

Jane Johnson, PhD

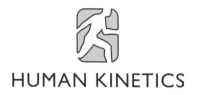

HUMAN KINETICS

Library of Congress Cataloging-in-Publication Data

Names: Johnson, Jane, 1965- author.
Title: Soft tissue therapy for the lower limb / Jane Johnson.
Other titles: Hands-on guides for therapists.
Description: Champaign, IL : Human Kinetics, [2025] | Series: Hands-on
  guides for therapists | Includes bibliographical references.
Identifiers: LCCN 2023059549 (print) | LCCN 2023059550 (ebook) | ISBN
  9781718215597 (paperback) | ISBN 9781718215603 (epub) | ISBN
  9781718215610 (pdf)
Subjects: MESH: Therapy, Soft Tissue--methods | Lower Extremity--physiology
  | BISAC: MEDICAL / Allied Health Services / Massage Therapy | MEDICAL /
  Alternative & Complementary Medicine
Classification: LCC R697.A4 (print) | LCC R697.A4 (ebook) | NLM WB 535 |
  DDC 610.73/7--dc23/eng/20240214
LC record available at https://lccn.loc.gov/2023059549
LC ebook record available at https://lccn.loc.gov/2023059550

ISBN: 978-1-7182-1559-7 (print)

Acquisitions Editor: Diana Vincer; **Developmental Editor:** Amy Stahl; **Managing Editor:** Hannah Werner; **Copyeditor:** Jenny MacKay; **Permissions Manager:** Laurel Mitchell; **Graphic Designer:** Denise Lowry; **Cover Designer:** Keri Evans; **Cover Design Specialist:** Susan Rothermel Allen; **Photograph (cover):** MICROGEN IMAGES/SCIENCE PHOTO LIBRARY/Getty Images; **Photographs (interior):** © Human Kinetics, unless otherwise noted; **Photo Production Manager:** Jason Allen; **Senior Art Manager:** Kelly Hendren; **Illustrations:** © Human Kinetics; **Printer:** Versa Press

Printed in the United States of America   10 9 8 7 6 5 4 3 2 1

The paper in this book is certified under a sustainable forestry program.

Human Kinetics
1607 N. Market Street
Champaign, IL 61820
USA

United States and International
Website: **US.HumanKinetics.com**
Email: info@hkusa.com
Phone: 1-800-747-4457

Canada
Website: **Canada.HumanKinetics.com**
Email: info@hkcanada.com

E8778

Contents

Series Preface

Massage may be one of the oldest therapies still used today. At present, more therapists than ever before are practising an ever-expanding range of massage techniques. Many of these techniques are taught through massage schools and within degree courses. Our need now is to provide the best clinical and educational resources that will enable massage therapists to learn the required techniques for delivering massage therapy to clients. Human Kinetics has developed the Hands-On Guides for Therapists series with this in mind.

The Hands-On Guides for Therapists series provides specific tools of assessment and treatment that fall within the realm of massage therapists but may also be useful for other bodyworkers, such as physical therapists, osteopaths, chiropractors, sports therapists and fitness instructors. Each book in the series is a step-by-step guide to delivering the techniques to clients. Each book features a full-colour interior packed with photos illustrating every technique. Tips provide handy advice to help you adjust your technique, and throughout each book are questions that enable you to test your knowledge and skill, which will be particularly helpful if you are attempting to pass a qualification exam. We've even provided the answers!

You might be using a book from the Hands-On Guides for Therapists series to obtain the required skills to help you pass a course or to brush up on skills you learned in the past. You might be a course tutor looking for new ways to make postural assessment or soft tissue techniques come alive with your students. This series provides easy-to-follow steps that will make the transition from theory to practice seem effortless. The Hands-On Guides for Therapists series is an essential resource for all those who are serious about massage therapy.

Preface

*S*oft Tissue Therapy for the Lower Limb is intended for use by professionals who use hands-on skills as part of their treatment. This book will help you to apply massage, stretching, soft tissue release (STR) and trigger point release techniques when working with clients with common lower limb conditions. It also includes a chapter on postural assessment of the lower limb (chapter 1) and three chapters on strengthening exercises (chapters 7-9 in part III). In this book, you will find specific information about which soft tissue techniques and strengthening exercises are appropriate for 31 different musculoskeletal conditions affecting the hips, buttocks, thighs, knees, legs, ankles and feet.

Part I focuses on assessment techniques and treatment outcomes. In chapter 1, you will learn how to assess lower limb posture from the anterior, posterior and lateral views, learning to identify, for example, lateral tilt of the pelvis, pelvic rotation, genu varum (bow-leggedness), genu valgum (knock knees), genu recurvatum (hyperextension of the knees), genu flexum (flexed knees), tibial torsion, pes valgus (ankle pronation), pes varus (ankle supination), pes planus (flatfootedness) and pes cavus (high arches), and the consequences of these postures on soft tissues. An appendix provides a handy lower limb postural assessment chart you can use to document your findings or to simply use as an aide-mémoire. Chapter 2 explains how to decide on an overall treatment plan by working with your client to set specific treatment goals and provides examples of how to do this. It is important that we can demonstrate the effectiveness of our treatments, and in this chapter, you will find tips on measuring pain, muscle length, joint range and everyday function.

Part II is divided into four chapters, each discussing common musculoskeletal conditions affecting a different part of the lower limb. This part of the book begins with chapter 3, discussing the gluteal, groin and hip flexor muscles. Chapter 4 covers the hamstrings and quadriceps and chapter 5, the knee, calf and shin, whilst conditions affecting the foot and ankle can be found in chapter 6. The pattern of information in these chapters is the same: for each condition, you will discover when it may be appropriate to use massage, trigger point release, STR and stretching. For conditions for which strengthening exercises are useful, you are directed to the relevant chapter later in the book. As part of recovery from a musculoskeletal condition, it is important that a person is as engaged as possible with their rehabilitation. For this reason, active STR, active stretches and active trigger point release techniques are included where relevant. Research into the effectiveness of hands-on techniques is limited. However, where a useful reference has been identified for a particular technique, this has been included along with a description of that source. The full list of references cited in the text can be found at the end of the book, organised by chapter.

In part III, the focus is on strengthening exercises – specifically, exercises that a person can perform safely with minimal equipment and without supervision. The chapters in this part of the book further reinforce the importance of a person's active engagement in their recovery. In this section, you will find exercises to help in the treatment of conditions affecting the hips (chapter 7), knees (chapter 8) and feet and ankles (chapter 9). To gauge the effectiveness of a strengthening programme, it is important to know which muscles are weak. Each of these chapters is organised the same way, beginning with how to test the strength of specific groups of muscles followed by suitable exercises to use if those muscles are found to be weak. Wherever possible, multiple testing positions are illustrated – standing, seated, supine, prone or side-lying – so that whatever the capacity of your client, you are certain to find a position that they find comfortable. Similarly, multiple different exercise positions are also shown. Wherever possible, exercises have been presented from those likely to be easiest to those likely to be more difficult, with explanations as to how to progress an exercise and for whom an exercise may be suitable. The aim of the information in this part of the book is to help people to regain their everyday function, and to that end, examples of functional exercises are also provided.

As with other titles in the Hands-On Guides for Therapists series, in *Soft Tissue Therapy for the Lower Limb*, you will find tips based on the author's many years of experience as a physiotherapist and soft tissue therapist, along with multiple photographs illustrating the techniques. Special thanks to Tim Allardyce from RehabMyPatient.com for kindly permitting use of his exercise images in chapters 7, 8 and 9.

Acknowledgements

This book has been made possible with the support of the team at Human Kinetics. Thank you to Jolynn Gower, the original acquisitions editor who accepted my idea for this title; to Diana Vincer, the acquisitions editor who took over the project; and to Amy Stahl, the developmental editor who joined Diana in providing support throughout the process. I would also like to thank the copyeditor, Jenny MacKay, for asking important clarifying questions. Thank you to the designer, Denise Lowry, for her essential role in bringing the book to life. I would like to do a shout-out to Barry Johnson, Human Kinetics' international sales director, and his team, including Lisa Lehnert, whose efforts have resulted in other titles in the Hands-On series being translated into multiple languages. It is wonderful that the information in this series is now available to therapists worldwide, and I have every confidence that Barry and his team will have equal success with this book too. Thank you also to the marketing implementation manager, Jenny Lokshin, and the marketing manager, Madeline Koenig-Schappe, for their roles in raising awareness of this title. I don't think I have ever seen a royalty accountant acknowledged, and I would like to rectify that. Tina Kinder has been my royalty accountant and, over the years, has diligently processed my royalties and answered my questions about them. I love sharing information, I love writing books and, of course, it's rather nice to get paid for it.

A very big thank you must go to Tim Allardyce, who generously let me use images from his online exercise prescription platform Rehab My Patient (www.rehabmypatient .com) and was extremely patient in the process of getting these implemented. You can find these wonderfully clear photos in chapters 7, 8 and 9.

PART I

Assessment Techniques and Treatment Outcomes

The first part of this book is all about assessment: how to assess a client's posture and how to perform tests that will later help you determine whether your treatment has been effective. Chapter 1 provides a step-by-step guide to postural assessment of the lower limb and teaches you what to look for when conducting an assessment from the anterior, posterior and lateral views. Chapter 2 explains how to use common muscle length and joint range of motion tests, pain and symptoms scores and functional assessment scales. These tests, scores and scales are valuable when used before and after treatment because they help determine whether your client has benefitted from, for example, an increase in muscle length, a reduction in pain or an improvement in function.

Postural Assessment of the Lower Limb

Learning Outcomes

After reading this chapter, you should be able to do the following:

- Assess a client for lateral tilt of the pelvis and pelvic rotation.
- Determine whether a client has genu varum or genu valgum knees.
- Describe at least one consequence of each of the lateral pelvic tilt, pelvic rotation, genu varum and genu valgum postures.
- Identify internal rotation of the femur and the consequences of this posture.
- Judge whether a client has a neutral, anteriorly tilted or posteriorly tilted pelvis and what might be the consequences of these postures.
- State what a person's stance and the shape and tone of their muscles might indicate.
- Identify the position of the knee and whether there is rotation of the lower limb, rotation of the tibia or both.
- Describe the consequences of rotation on the lower limb, knee or tibia.
- Explain how to measure the Q angle.
- Determine whether a person has a neutral, genu recurvatum or genu flexum knee posture.
- Recognise pes valgus and pes varus ankle postures.
- Identify pes planus and pes cavus foot postures.

This chapter contains three sections that provide detailed information about the kinds of things you might observe when conducting a postural assessment of the lower limb. It does not matter in which order you carry out the assessment – whether you start with an anterior (front), posterior (back) or lateral (side) view – but it is helpful to be systematic in your approach so as not to miss anything. You may find the lower limb postural assessment chart in the appendix useful. Try not to jump to conclusions about what your observations mean. To form an opinion as to what might be the problem and what kind of treatment might be most helpful, document your findings and use these together with the subjective history you take from your client and any other tests you perform. This is important because the postural assessment alone provides only some of the information required to help you formulate a treatment plan. For example, it will not tell you about the range of movement in a joint, the strength of muscles or how a lower limb problem is affecting a person's function. A postural assessment does, however, provide clues that can be invaluable for eliciting further information from the client. The anatomical consequences of many of the postures are detailed in the sections that follow.

Once you have gained an overview of the client's stance, turn your attention to more specific items, such as whether any muscles appear to be atrophied (thinner and wasted) or hypertrophied (larger and bulkier). Next, consider each part of the lower limbs: the pelvis, knees, ankles and feet. Examine these in more detail, observing their position and shape and whether there is evidence of injury (bruising), surgery (scars) or an underlying condition (swelling, skin discolouration, varicose veins). Finally, remember to always record whether a person walks with an aid or uses a supportive device, such as a knee brace or foot orthotic.

Throughout this chapter, you will find tables detailing whether a muscle is likely to be shortened or lengthened in each specific posture. This is useful because one of your treatment goals might be to lengthen a shortened muscle or to shorten a lengthened one.

Anterior View

Stance

Take an overview of how your client stands. Do they naturally stand with their legs together, or are they more comfortable with a wide stance? Consider the foot position and weight distribution (see figure 1.1). Do they look comfortable as they stand? Are they happy to place their weight equally through both legs, or do they appear to favour one leg more than the other? If so, why might that be? Are they recovering from a recent injury or operation, or could this be a habit they have developed due to a previous problem? Do they need the support of an aid, such as a stick, crutch, knee brace or ankle brace? Do the lower limbs appear to be shaped the same, or is there evidence of genu varum (bow-leggedness) or genu valgum (knock knees)? (You can read more about how to identify genu varum and valgum and the consequences of these postures later in this section.)

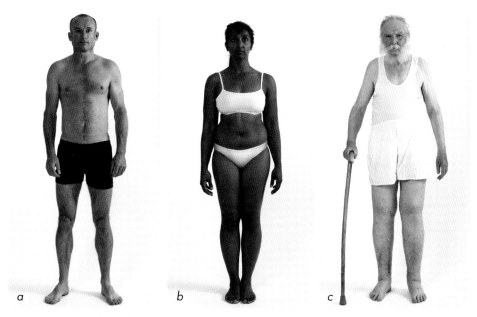

a   b   c

Figure 1.1   Examples of *(a)* wide, *(b)* narrow and *(c)* supported stances.
Courtesy of Emma Kelly Photography.

TIP

If you notice your client is standing in a wide stance, ask them to stand with their feet together (so the medial malleoli of the ankles are as close as possible), if you believe it is safe to do so. Ask how they feel. Clients with weak adductor muscles of the hip may dislike this position and feel particularly unbalanced. You can get a sense of this yourself by standing with your feet together. Notice your adductors contracting to keep you in this position.

Consequences

Clients who stand in a wide stance create a wide base of support for themselves. Why might they do this? Is it because they feel unbalanced? Could it be that in some cases they have weak hip adductor muscles relative to their abductor muscles?

Anterior View

Lateral Tilt of the Pelvis

The pelvis is laterally tilted when one side is higher than the other. This posture is sometimes called 'hip hitch' because the pelvis has been hitched up on one side. The illustration shown in figure 1.2 has been deliberately exaggerated to show a pelvis that is tilted upwards on the right. In reality, it is more common to see a subtle shift, as in figure 1.3. The amount of pelvic tilt shown in the photograph may not at first be apparent, but if you observe this man's left knee and left hand, you will see that these are both lower than the right knee and right hand.

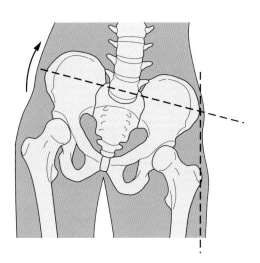

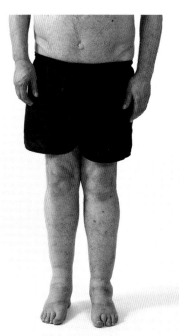

Figure 1.2   Exaggerated to show the pelvis tilted upwards on the right.

Figure 1.3   Pelvis laterally tilted on the client's right side.

Courtesy of Emma Kelly Photography.

TIP

When you are first using anterior postural assessment, it is easy to confuse a person's left and right. Remember that the right side of the photograph in figure 1.3 is the man's *left* side; the left side of the photograph is the man's *right* side.

TIP

To experience what a laterally tilted pelvis feels like, stand in front of a mirror, with both feet on the floor. Imagine that you have your leg in a cast and cannot flex at the knee. Place your hands on your hips and slowly lift the heel of your right foot off the floor, but keep the toes of your right foot on the floor as you do this. You can see and feel the right side of your pelvis as it rises and as you laterally flex to the right at your lumbar spine to accommodate this position.

Consequences

Table 1.1 lists the muscle lengths associated with a laterally tilted pelvis. For example, to compensate for a pelvis that is raised on the right, a client may have increased lateral flexion of the lumbar spine (to the right), which may correspond with the appearance of more or deeper skin creases on the right. In this case, the right quadratus lumborum muscle may be shorter, as may some of the right lumbar erector spinae muscles. The hip joints are affected also. The right hip is adducted, whereas the left hip is abducted. Therefore, a client may have a pelvis raised on the right with shortened hip abductors on the left and shortened adductor muscles on the right.

Table 1.1   Muscle Lengths Associated With a Laterally Tilted Pelvis

	Pelvis raised on the right	Pelvis raised on the left
Lumbar spine	Flexed to the right; concave on the right	Flexed to the left; concave on the left
Lumbar muscles	Shortened right quadratus lumborum and right lumbar erector spinae	Shortened left quadratus lumborum and left lumbar erector spinae
Effects on the hip joint	Right hip is adducted; left hip is abducted	Left hip is adducted; right hip is abducted
Effects on the muscles of the hip	Shortening of right hip adductors and left hip abductors; imbalance between the left and right hamstrings	Shortening of left hip adductors and right hip abductors; imbalance between the left and right hamstrings

Anterior View

Pelvic Rotation

Imagine the pelvis can rotate with respect to the spine in the way that a bead can rotate with respect to a string. A good way to determine whether your client has a rotated pelvis is to examine the position of the anterior superior iliac spines (ASIS). When the pelvis is rotated clockwise, the client's left ASIS will be closer to you and the right ASIS will move away from you. When the pelvis is rotated anticlockwise, the client's right ASIS will be closer to you and the left ASIS farther away. The illustrations in figure 1.4 exaggerate rotator movements; in reality, they are far more subtle.

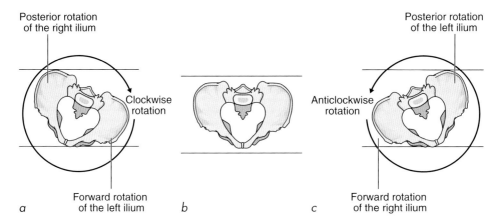

Figure 1.4 Pelvic rotation with *(a)* clockwise rotation, *(b)* no rotation and *(c)* anticlockwise rotation.

TIP

To determine pelvic rotation, it helps to imagine that the client is standing between two sheets of glass, one in front and one behind. Does the ASIS on one side of the pelvis appear to be closer to the glass behind the client than that on the other side?

Consequences

If the pelvis is rotated away from you on the left (clockwise), the right internal oblique and left external oblique may be shortened. If the client has a pelvis rotated forwards to the right (anticlockwise), the opposite may be true. Pelvic rotation has a corkscrewing effect on the entire body. The result is that muscles and joints throughout the body are affected, including the feet (see figure 1.5).

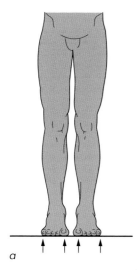 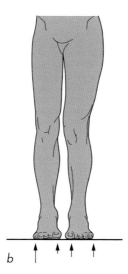 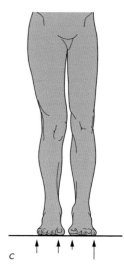

a   b   c

Figure 1.5 *(a)* Neutral pelvis with both anterior superior iliac spines aligned. Knees face forwards. There is equal pressure beneath the medial and lateral sides of the foot. *(b)* The whole pelvis is rotated to the right. Knees no longer face forwards. There is increased pressure on the lateral side of the right foot. *(c)* The whole pelvis is rotated to the left. Knees no longer face forwards. There is increased pressure on the lateral side of the left foot.

TIP

Table 1.2 sets out the effect of pelvic rotation on the feet. You can easily test the effect pelvic rotation has on the feet by rotating to the left and right and feeling what happens to the contact points of the soles of your feet with the floor.

Table 1.2 Pelvic Rotation and Its Effect on the Feet

ROTATION OF THE PELVIS TO THE LEFT	
Left foot	**Right foot**
• Increased supination	• Increased pronation
• There is increased pressure on the lateral side of the foot and decreased pressure on the medial side of the foot as a result of increased inversion of the forefoot	• The pressure is roughly equal on the lateral and medial sides of the foot

ROTATION OF THE PELVIS TO THE RIGHT	
Left foot	**Right foot**
• Increased pronation	• Increased supination
• The pressure is roughly equal on the lateral and medial sides of the foot	• There is increased pressure on the lateral side of the foot and decreased pressure on the medial side of the foot as a result of increased inversion of the forefoot

Anterior View

Muscle Bulk and Tone

Compare muscle bulk (figure 1.6a) and the tone of the left and right thighs. Does the girth of each thigh appear equal? Would you agree that the region of the vastus medialis on this client appears hypertrophied on his right thigh compared to his left (figure 1.6b)?

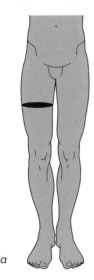
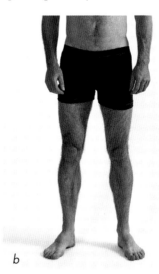

a   b

Figure 1.6   Assessing the girth of the thigh muscles *(a)* to determine if they are the same or *(b)* whether there is any hypertrophy.

Photo *b* courtesy of Emma Kelly Photography.

TIP

Shadows falling on the limbs can make it difficult to determine whether there is any asymmetry in muscle bulk. If in doubt, either change the light source or move your client slightly to help determine whether what you are observing is indeed atrophy or hypertrophy or simply shadow.

Consequences

An increase in bulk suggests increased use or weight bearing on that side of the body, whereas atrophy of muscles (in a healthy person) suggests disuse. Atrophy in muscles of the lower limb is common after immobilisation of the limb or a prolonged period of bed rest. Atrophy in a muscle will result in decreased strength in that muscle. If this occurs in one thigh only, there will be imbalance, and this can lead to additional stressors on the muscles and joints of the opposite leg.

Anterior View

Genu Varum (Bow-Leggedness)

Next, let's look at the knees. Genu varum, popularly termed *bow legs* because the lower limbs take on the shape of an archer's bow, is misalignment of the knee joint. Ask your client to stand with the feet together, the medial malleoli as close together as possible. Observe the distance of the medial femoral condyles and their distance from an imaginary plumb line. If one knee appears to be farther from the midline and the overall limb has taken on a bowlike appearance, this is evidence of genu varum (figure 1.7a). Genu varum affects both the knee joint itself and the muscles supporting it. Osteoarthritic changes or degradation of menisci may be more likely to occur on the side of the knee subject to greater compressive forces. Overstretching of soft tissues is likely on the opposite side of the knee. In this posture, there is gapping of the lateral aspect of the knee and increased tension on the lateral collateral ligament as well as compression of the medial meniscus (figure 1.7b).

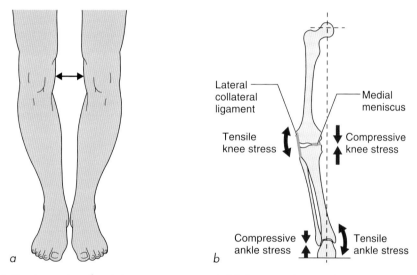

Figure 1.7 Assessing for (a) genu varum and (b) the gapping and compressive forces in this posture.

TIP

If you are the sort of person who likes to quantify posture, you may be interested to know that the typical angle formed between the anatomical axis of the femur and the anatomical axis of the tibia on the medial side of the knee is approximately 195 degrees (Levangie and Norkin 2001). In the genu varum knee posture, the medial tibiofemoral angle is less than 180 degrees.

Consequences

In the genu varum posture (figure 1.7a), there is increased tensile stress on the lateral side of the knee and medial side of the ankle and increased compressive force on the medial side of the knee and lateral side of the ankle (figure 1.7b). A way to appreciate the consequence of these strains is to imagine the gapping motion that has occurred in the lateral aspect of the knee joint. Gapping means that the lateral collateral knee ligament is tensed and possibly weakened, providing less stability and increasing the likelihood of lateral collateral ligament injury. The medial meniscus is compressed, possibly causing damage there too.

The mechanical axis of the knee is vertical, meaning that during typical bilateral weight bearing, forces are transmitted through the centre of the knee joint and distributed equally through the medial and lateral compartments. Malalignment of the joint shifts the transition of force to the medial aspect of the knee, which affects balance and gait and may predispose a client to knee pathology. For example, some studies have found that knee malalignment is associated with higher rates of knee osteoarthritis (McWilliams et al. 2010). Whether a joint's pathology progresses to severe osteoarthritis depends on its existing state of vulnerability: A joint with mild osteoarthritis, for example, may be less vulnerable to the biomechanical effects of malalignment than a more damaged joint (Cerejo et al. 2002). If you imagine the mechanical axis in figure 1.7b as a bowstring, you can see how the genu varum posture gets its nickname and how it has a tendency to worsen. People with osteoarthritis who demonstrate this posture often report knee pain.

As you can see from table 1.3, in the genu varum posture, certain muscles are lengthened and others are shortened; you can see that the iliotibial band is tensed and lengthened compared to a neutral posture, as is the biceps femoris, whereas the gracilis and semitendinosus are shortened. This may have little impact on day-to-day activities but could compromise a client's participation in sport, for example.

Additionally, not only does the genu varum posture shorten the quadriceps, it also affects the direction of pull by the quadriceps on the patella. There may be a tendency for the patella to be pulled medially. The direction of pull of the patella is important for overall knee stability; altering the direction could disrupt this bone's normal gliding mechanism and lead to instability of the knee. In extreme cases, the genu varum posture could contribute to degenerative changes in the patellofemoral joint.

Postural bow legs occur as a result of medial rotation of the femur and pronation of the foot (Kendall, McCreary, and Provance 1993). The atypical joint position is also likely to affect the normal glide and roll of the femur on the tibia that occurs during flexion and extension movements of the knee. During weight bearing, there may be medial rotation of the leg, and in turn, the medial side of the foot can be elevated from the floor unless compensatory subtalar pronation occurs. Other compensatory movement may include eversion of the talus and pronation of the intertarsal joints as a means of regaining contact with the ground surface. This posture adversely affects balance and is significant especially in the older population, in which genu varum is more common, as are falls. Genu varum deformity has been shown to increase neutral postural sway in the mediolateral direction and increase risk of falls (Samaei et al. 2012).

Table 1.3 Muscle Lengths Associated With Genu Varum Knee Posture

Area	Shortened muscles	Lengthened muscles
Thigh	Quadriceps Internal hip rotators Gracilis Semitendinosus and semimembrano- sus relative to biceps femoris	Lateral rotators of the hip Biceps femoris relative to semitendi- nosus and semimembranosus
Leg	Fibular (peroneal) muscles	Popliteus Tibialis posterior Long toe flexors

Anterior View

Genu Valgum (Knock Knees)

This posture is assessed by asking your client to stand with their medial femoral condyles touching. Observe the distance of the medial malleoli from the midline (figure 1.8). If one ankle appears to be farther from the midline, this is evidence of genu valgum. As with genu varum, this knee posture affects both the knee joint itself and the muscles supporting it. Osteoarthritic changes or degradation of the meniscus may be more likely to occur on the side of the knee subject to greater compressive forces; overstretching of soft tissues is likely on the opposite side of the knee (figure 1.8b).

An increase in the valgus angle of the knee often coincides with leg-length discrepancy. It occurs on the side where the leg is longer, and there is also posterior pelvic torsion of the ilium on that side (Cooperstein and Lew 2009).

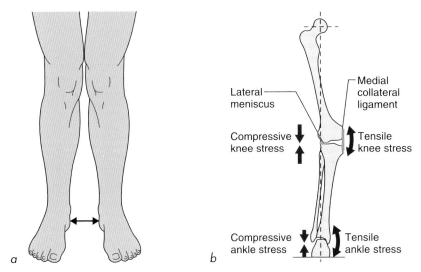

Figure 1.8 Assessing for (a) genu valgum and (b) the gapping and compressive forces in this posture.

TIP

As you learned in the section about the genu varum posture, the typical angle formed between the anatomical axis of the femur and the anatomical axis of the tibia on the medial side of the knee is approximately 195 degrees (Levangie and Norkin 2001). In the genu valgum knee posture, the medial tibiofemoral angle is greater than 195 degrees.

Consequences

In the genu valgum posture, there is increased tensile stress on the medial side of the knee and ankle and increased compressive force on the lateral side of the knee and ankle. People with this posture commonly report pain, though it cannot be assumed that this is due to the posture itself.

In this posture, there is gapping of the medial aspect of the knee, with increased tension in the medial collateral ligament, which could become weakened, providing less stability for the knee and increasing the likelihood of medial collateral ligament injury. The lateral meniscus is compressed, possibly causing damage there too.

During typical bilateral weight bearing, forces are transmitted through the centre of the knee joint and distributed equally through the medial and lateral compartments. In the genu valgum posture, force is shifted to the lateral aspect of the knee and could affect balance and gait. Altered joint mechanics may predispose a patient to knee pathology. Malalignment is associated with higher rates of knee osteoarthritis (McWilliams et al. 2010).

The gracilis, semitendinosus and sartorius are all lengthened and tensed. The tensor fasciae latae and the iliotibial band are compressed, as are tissues of the lateral leg compartment (see table 1.4).

The atypical joint position is also likely to affect the normal glide and roll of the femur on the tibia that occur during flexion and extension movements of the knee. There may also be a tendency for the patella to be pulled laterally, which could disrupt this bone's usual gliding mechanism. Together, these altered joint mechanics are likely to compromise knee function. In extreme cases, the genu valgum posture could contribute to degenerative changes in the patellofemoral joint. Proprioception is likely to be altered, which could affect balance.

Genu valgum is associated with postural change in other joints. This includes lumbar spine rotation on the contralateral side and excessive adduction and medial rotation of the hip, lateral tibial torsion, inversion of the talus, supination of the subtalar joints or intertarsal joints and pes planus (Riegger-Krugh and Keysor 1996).

Table 1.4 Muscle Lengths Associated With Genu Valgum Knee Posture

Area	Shortened muscles	Lengthened muscles
Thigh	Biceps femoris relative to semimembranosus and semitendinosus Tensor fasciae latae Hip adductors	Gracilis Semimembranosus and semitendinosus relative to biceps femoris Sartorius
Leg	Fibular (peroneal) muscles	

Anterior View

Patellar Position

The patella should be positioned in line with the tibial tuberosity. Observing the position of the patella does not reveal how it moves; therefore, this part of the anterior assessment is a good example of why it is important to also assess a person's function (see chapter 2) in addition to carrying out an assessment of their posture. It is nevertheless important to observe the position of the patella, because this can provide a clue as to whether maltracking of this bone is likely. Does it sit over the centre of the knee joint, or is it resting laterally (figure 1.9a) or medially (figure 1.9b)? Another question you might ask yourself is whether the patellae seem to sit neutrally or whether they appear compressed and tilting against the knee joints. People who stand with their knees hyperextended cause the patellae to be compressed, and although hyperextension is best examined from a lateral view, it is still possible to get a sense of whether the patellae rest comfortably against the tibiofemoral joints or whether they appear squashed against the joints due to hyperextension.

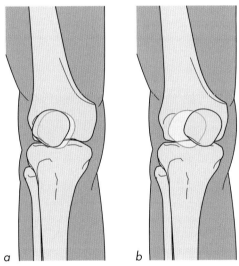

a   b

Figure 1.9   A right knee with *(a)* lateral maltracking and *(b)* medial maltracking.

TIP

One way to assess whether the patellae are compressed when performing an anterior view assessment is to imagine each knee is the headlight of a car. Imagine where the beam of that light might fall on the ground in front of the client. Do both beams hit at the same distance from the client? Where a patella is compressed, as in hyperextension of the knee, the beam will hit the floor closer on that side than the beam of the opposite knee (unless there is hyperextension of both joints). An illustration of how this might appear when viewing the knees posteriorly can be found in the section on posterior assessment.

Consequences

Because the patella is housed within the quadriceps tendon, and this in turn is housed in fascia connected to other structures, could an increase in tension in the muscles or the fascia of the medial or lateral sides of the knee (or both) contribute to maltracking (see table 1.5)? For example, could lateral maltracking be due to increased tension in the lateral retinaculum of the knee and the iliotibial band? Could medial maltracking be due to increased tension in the vastus medialis? Maltracking of the patella could potentially lead to pain and subluxation of that bone, disrupting typical function of the knee. Anterior knee pain can sometimes be explained by patellae tilting such that their inferior poles stick into the fat pad beneath the knee, a condition perhaps aggravated by forced or prolonged knee extension.

Table 1.5 Possible Consequences of Soft Tissue Tension in the Lateral and Medial Aspects of the Knee on Patella Tracking

Area of soft tissue tension	Lateral retinaculum of the knee Iliotibial band	Vastus medialis
Possible consequence	Lateral maltracking of the patella	Medial maltracking of the patella

Anterior View

Rotation of the Lower Limb

Assessing for rotation of the lower limb is the first step in helping to identify whether there is tibial torsion or rotation of the hip or femur. In a neutral position, the patella should point straight ahead with respect to the tibiofemoral joint. This means that if a client stands with the feet turned out slightly, as might be expected, the patella will also face outwards slightly but should still be aligned over the joint. Therefore, begin by observing the knee to get a general feel for whether it is in a neutral position or whether it is internally or externally rotated (figure 1.10).

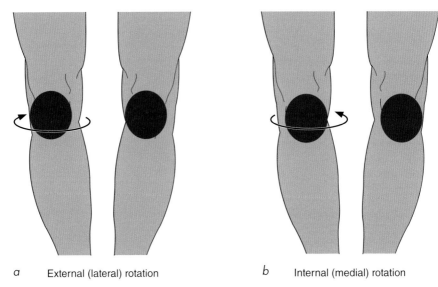

| a | External (lateral) rotation | b | Internal (medial) rotation |

Figure 1.10 Circles approximate the position of the kneecap and represent *(a)* external and *(b)* internal rotation of the knee.

TIP

Standing in front of a full-length mirror, turn both of your feet outwards, rotating the entire lower limb externally, and notice the position of your patellae. In this position, the femurs, knees and tibiae are externally rotated as a group. Next, reverse the position and stand pigeon-toed, rotating both lower limbs internally so that your feet are pointing inwards. Again, notice what happens to your patellae in this exaggerated posture. In this stance, the femurs, knees and tibiae are all internally rotated as a group.

Consequences

Because the femur and tibia attach at the knee joint, and this joint permits a small amount of rotation, it is possible for each bone to rotate in a different direction with respect to one another, and this can cause tibial torsion. You can read about tibial torsion in the next section, and you can read about an internally rotated femur as part of the posterior postural assessment.

Anterior View

Tibial Torsion

After assessing the position of the knee, it is helpful to consider whether there is any tibial torsion. In a clinical setting, tibial torsion tends to refer to torsion of the leg (i.e., rotation between the tibia and femur at the knee joint and movement between the tibia and talus at the ankle joint). Whether torsion is pure (within the bone itself, irrespective of joints) or clinical (longitudinal rotation about the leg due to lower limb joint positions), it is difficult to identify purely from postural assessment. A good starting point is to observe your client from the front and to note where the tibial tuberosities lie. Are they facing forwards and symmetrical, or does one face inwards (internal tibial torsion) or outwards (external tibial torsion)? Observe the position of the feet. Internal tibial torsion is associated with a toe-in posture and external torsion with a toe-out posture.

However, a patient can appear to have neutral tibiae when in fact they have torsion. An example is in figure 1.11. At first glance, the patient's legs appear neutral because her left and right tibial tuberosities are facing forwards, but observe her right knee, which does not face forwards. This indicates internal rotation of the femur. With internal rotation of the femur, you would expect to also have in-toeing, yet the client's feet are facing forwards. For the feet to face forwards, the tibia must have torsion *externally*.

> **TIP**
>
> A way of testing whether there is external rotation is to ask your client to stand so that the knees are facing forwards, if able. When a patient with external tibial torsion stands with the knees facing forwards, the external tibial torsion will be much more marked because the feet will have been placed in a marked toe-out position.

Although not all studies agree, some have found that torsion varies between the left and right legs within the same individual, with greater outward rotation of the right leg compared to the left (Clementz 1988; Mullaji et al. 2008). The reasons for this are not clear.

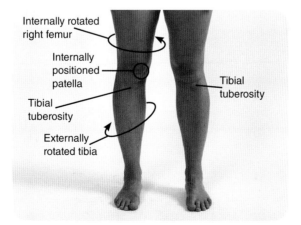

Figure 1.11 Patient with external tibial torsion of the right leg, which at first glance appears neutral.

Photo courtesy of Emma Kelly Photography.

Consequences

During walking, the pelvis rotates about the weight-bearing hip joint, with the pelvis on the side of the swinging leg moving forward. Various segments of the leg rotate in the same direction as the pelvis and in phase with pelvic rotation. The amplitude of rotation increases proximally to distally, with the tibia rotating about its long axis three times as much as the pelvis rotates (Inman 1966). Rotation of this kind is a typical part of gait; excessive internal or external rotation will adversely affect these biomechanics and therefore is likely to increase the energy expenditure of walking.

Some muscles can affect joints they do not cross. The mechanisms for this are unclear but are likely to include the interconnectedness of muscles synchronised via the fascial system. The gluteal muscles and soleus can each affect both the hip and the knee joints. Excessive tibial torsion has been found to reduce the capacity of these muscles and, as a result, diminish hip and knee extension during gait (Hicks et al. 2007).

Certain sports might aggravate this posture. For example, golfers develop postures throughout their bodies that are associated with rotation, including in the joints of the lower limbs and in the soft tissues associated with these joints. The pivoting movement inherent to golf increases the likelihood of tibial torsion on the leg that remains static. For example, moving the club to the right at the start of a swing and rotating the upper body clockwise to the right produce internal rotation of the left hip and internal torsion on the right leg, which is fixed to the ground.

Torsion of the tibia alters the position of the meniscus with respect to the femur and the direction of pull of the patella. Ultimately, this affects how forces are transmitted through the knee joint. These could be reasons why tibial torsion is associated with early-onset arthritis, patellofemoral arthritis, genu valgum and genu varum. Malalignment of the knee joint could increase the risk of knee injury.

Clinical tibial torsion also affects the feet and ankles (see table 1.6). Lateral tibial torsion is associated with a toe-out foot position and increased supination, heel inversion and accentuation of the medial longitudinal arch. Medial tibial torsion is associated with a toe-in foot position, which can lead to tripping or feeling clumsy when walking. There is increased subtalar pronation, the heel is everted and the medial longitudinal arch is decreased. These changes may cause pain, reduce balance and affect gait. Atypical joint positions in the foot and ankle are likely to impair sporting performance, and in some cases, they could contribute to early joint degeneration, especially in sports or occupations involving repeated high impact. In a study of 836 patients, Turner and Smillie (1981) found that external torsion of the tibia was correlated with lesions of the extensor apparatus, notably in patients with unstable patellofemoral joints and Osgood-Schlatter disease. It was not known whether these conditions led to the development of increased external tibial torsion or whether pre-existing increased tibial torsion predisposed the patients to subsequent development of patellofemoral instability and Osgood-Schlatter disease. By contrast, patients with inverted feet (associated with internal tibial torsion) have an advantage when running distances of 15 to 20 metres (16-22 yd), because this posture promotes short, rapid steps, theoretically because tibial torsion shortens the hamstrings, limiting a wider step. Thus, there is greater ground contact whilst moving, and this may improve dynamic balance (Bloomfield, Ackland, and Elliott 1994).

Because tibial torsion can affect and be affected by movements in the pelvis, hip, foot and ankle, there may be imbalance in muscles throughout the entire lower limb, and these will be highly individualised. Muscles shown in table 1.7 provide a guide only. Because of the small degree of rotational movement involved in tibial torsion, there are few significant changes to the length of muscles in this posture. Joint position and the effect on ligaments and articular structures may be of greater significance than muscle lengths. It is likely that many structures contribute to the checking of knee rotation, including the cruciate ligaments, collateral ligaments, posteromedial capsule, posterolateral capsule, popliteus tendon and menisci distorted in the direction of the corresponding femoral condyle (Levangie and Norkin 2001). These structures will be affected when there is an increase in torsion involving joints (rather than pure torsion within the tibia). The degree of change in the muscles listed in table 1.7 may be minor and is included only to show that some change is likely to occur, as when, for example, the distal attachments of the hamstrings are reorientated as the tibia rotates either internally or externally.

Table 1.6   Tibial Torsion and Corresponding Changes in the Foot

	Lateral tibial torsion	Medial tibial torsion
Foot position	Toe-out	Toe-in
Foot changes	Increased subtalar supination Inversion of heel Accentuation of medial longitudinal arch	Increased subtalar pronation Eversion of heel Decrease in medial longitudinal arch

Table 1.7   Muscle Lengths Associated With Increased Tibial Torsion

Direction of torsion	Shortened muscles	Lengthened muscles
External tibial torsion	Biceps femoris relative to semitendinosus and semimembranosus Iliotibial band Sartorius Muscles and ligaments associated with pronation of the foot	Semitendinosus and semimembranosus relative to biceps femoris Popliteus Muscles and ligaments associated with pronation of the foot
Internal tibial torsion	Semitendinosus and semimembranosus relative to the biceps femoris Popliteus Muscles and ligaments associated with supination of the foot	Biceps femoris relative to semitendinosus and semimembranosus Iliotibial band Sartorius Muscles and ligaments associated with supination of the foot

Measuring Tibial Torsion

True tibial torsion is the twisting of the tibia within the bone itself around its longitudinal axis. With respect to the proximal end, the distal end of the tibia is twisted laterally

(continued)

Measuring Tibial Torsion (continued)

and contributes to the toe-out posture observed in typical standing. There is no agreed norm for the degree of twist, because studies have used different proximal and distal end points on the tibia when making measurements. One method of measurement is to take either magnetic resonance imaging or computed tomography scans of the proximal (figure 1.12a) and distal (figure 1.12b) ends of the tibia, just below and above the articulating surfaces, respectively, then draw lines bisecting each scan image. The tibial torsion angle is the angle formed by the bisecting lines (figure 1.12c).

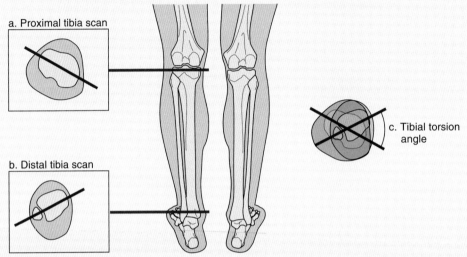

Figure 1.12 One method for calculating true tibial torsion, using the left leg as an example. *(a)* Proximal tibia scan, just below the articulating surface (note the absence of the fibula at this point of the cross-section). *(b)* Distal tibia scan, just above the articulating surface (the fibula is present at this level of the cross-section and can be seen as the smaller bone). *(c)* Tibial torsion angle.

In their review of nine studies carried out between 1909 and 1975, Turner and Smillie (1981) reported tibial torsion measurements ranging from 14 to 23 degrees but noted that different measuring devices were used, making comparison difficult. In a more recent study, Strecker and colleagues (1997) recorded torsion in 504 typical tibiae as 34.9 ± 15.9 degrees. Levangie and Norkin (2001) suggested using the figure of 20 to 30 degrees for tibial torsion in the general population.

Assessing tibial torsion before treatment is a challenge. Not only are there differences in the degree of tibial torsion between different studies, but different degrees of torsion have been found between the left and right tibiae of the same patient (Gandhi et al. 2014; Strecker et al. 1997) and amongst ethnic groups. For example, Mullaji and colleagues (2008) recorded tibial torsion of only 21.6 ± 7.6 degrees in 100 limbs in a study of non-arthritic Indian adults and suggested that the variation between groups could be due to culture-specific sitting postures. For example, Japanese people traditionally sit on the floor in knee flexion, with the feet turned inwards and the buttocks resting on the feet, exerting an *internal* force on the tibia, whereas sitting cross-legged, as is common in some Indian populations (the lotus position in yoga), increases *external* tibial rotation.

Anterior View

Q Angle

The Q angle describes the relationships between the pelvis, leg and foot. It measures the angle between the rectus femoris quadriceps muscle – hence, the name *Q angle* – and the patellar tendon (see figure 1.13). It is useful because, theoretically, it may help predict the likelihood of some types of knee problems, and as such, it may indicate the need for prophylactic treatment. To determine the Q angle of a client, follow these steps with the client standing:

1. Find the midpoint of the patella.
2. From this point, draw a line running longitudinally up the femur to the anterior superior iliac spine (ASIS).
3. Find the tibial tuberosity.
4. Draw a line from the midpoint of the patella to the tibial tuberosity. Extend this line superior to the patella, thus creating an angle with your first line.

The angle between these two lines is the Q angle and is usually around 15 to 20 degrees, but it varies between males and females and amongst individuals.

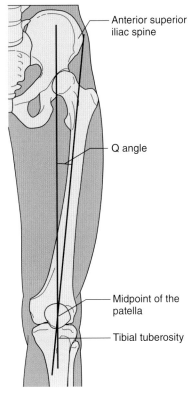

Figure 1.13 The Q angle.

Labels: Anterior superior iliac spine; Q angle; Midpoint of the patella; Tibial tuberosity

TIP

It is more accurate to measure the Q angle of a client when they are standing than supine, because when a client is standing, the patella is under the usual weight-bearing stresses.

Consequences

As a result of a wider pelvis, women have a greater Q angle than men do. It has been postulated that when the Q angle is greater than typical, the client might experience greater stress through the patella when performing repetitive exercises that rely on the use of the knee. This could lead to maltracking of the patella so that it does not glide smoothly on the femoral grooves, which in turn could lead to microtrauma. Over time, this microtrauma could develop into more serious pathology, such as degradation of the patellofemoral cartilage.

Clients with increased pronation of the foot may have an atypical Q angle, perhaps as a result of internal rotation of the tibia. If this rotation is prolonged, the alteration in usual biomechanics could result in increased stress on the knee joint. This in turn could lead to more serious knee problems. It is important to remember, however, that an atypical Q angle does not mean that a client will definitely experience knee problems.

Anterior View

Ankles

When observing the ankles, the medial malleoli should be level with each other, and the lateral malleoli should be level with each other. Look also to see whether any swelling or discolouration is evident. Do you observe any eversion or inversion? In other words, does the client appear to be rolling in onto the medial side of the foot, or rolling out with greater pressure on the outside of the foot and an increased space between the medial side of the foot and the floor? Figure 1.14 demonstrates how postural assessment can help provide important information about injuries to the lower limb, in this example, to the ankle.

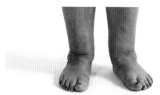

Figure 1.14 The ankles of the person shown here demonstrate how childhood musculo-skeletal injuries can have lifelong effects. This 74-year-old woman fractured her left ankle very badly as a young girl. Can you see, from the anterior view, that the ankle appears to have rolled inwards on the medial side, with loss of the arch?

Courtesy of Emma Kelly Photography.

TIP

The ankle inversion posture is not common. Therefore, if you can see a gap between the underside of your client's foot in the region of the medial arch, this could simply mean that they have a high arch and not that their foot is inverted.

Consequences

Please refer to the sections on pes valgus and pes varus of the posterior postural assessment for a full description of what changes in the position of the malleoli might mean.

Anterior View

Foot Position

In typical standing, the feet turn outwards slightly by about 6 to 8 degrees (figure 1.15). How has your client positioned their feet? The feet should be turned out to the same angle, equidistant from an imaginary plumb line.

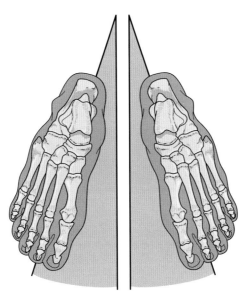

Figure 1.15 Common foot position.

TIP

If you observe asymmetry in the foot positions or the feet are not positioned as in figure 1.15, ask your client to take a few steps forwards and backwards and then reassess them. If they return to the same foot position, then this is likely to be the typical foot position for them.

Consequences

Feet turned out in a ballet-type stance could result from external rotation at the hip joint, lateral tibial torsion or both. External hip rotation could indicate shortening of the gluteus maximus and the posterior fibres of the gluteus medius, along with the iliotibial band. A client who stands with their feet turned inwards (pigeon-toed) may have shortened internal rotators of the hip, a medially rotated tibia or both. Table 1.8 summarises this information.

Table 1.8 Changes Associated With Toe-Out and Toe-In Foot Positions

	Toe-out position	Toe-in position
Possible position of the hip joint	Externally rotated	Internally rotated
Possible position of the tibia	Lateral tibial torsion	Medial tibial torsion
Muscles that might be shortened	External rotators of the femur; iliotibial band	Internal rotators of the femur

Anterior View

Other Observations

Finally, note anything else that you have not yet documented. Pay particular attention to swelling around the joints, skin discolouration and scars. In the photograph in figure 1.16a, can you see the increase in tension in the tendon of the person's right tibialis anterior muscle? It could have been that they were correcting postural sway just as this photograph was taken, or they could have a significant difference between the tendons of this muscle on their left and right legs. Noting your observations regarding the client's toes can also be helpful. The ankles and feet of the client in figure 1.16b appear swollen, and the second toe of the right foot is squashed, potentially causing pain or affecting gait.

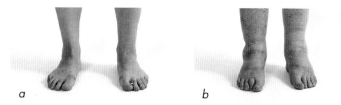

Figure 1.16 *(a)* Tension in the right tibialis anterior muscle; *(b)* an example of ankle and foot swelling and a squashed toe.

Courtesy of Emma Kelly Photography.

Posterior View

Pelvic Rim

Lateral tilt of the pelvis was discussed in the anterior view section of this chapter and can also be assessed posteriorly. A good way to check whether the pelvis is level when you are new to postural assessment is to sit or crouch down behind your client and gently place your hands on their waist. Press first into the fleshy part of the waist and then down onto the bony iliac crests, or the pelvic rim (figure 1.17). Gauge whether the left and right sides of the pelvis feel level.

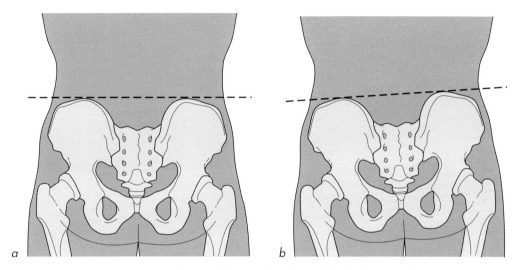

a   b

Figure 1.17 *(a)* A neutral pelvis and *(b)* a pelvis laterally tilted upwards to the right.

TIP

To help you visualise the effect a laterally tilted pelvis has on the hips, picture the pelvis as a tabletop with two table legs beneath it (Levangie and Norkin 2001) (figure 1.18). The legs are free to swing left and right (i.e., to abduct or adduct). Now imagine tilting the tabletop down to the left (up to the right). What happens to the table legs? They will continue to hang down perpendicularly, but notice what has happened to the angles they now form with the tabletop (representing the attachment of the femur at the hip). The right leg is adducted (the internal angle has decreased), and the left leg is abducted (the external angle has increased).

(continued)

TIP *(continued)*

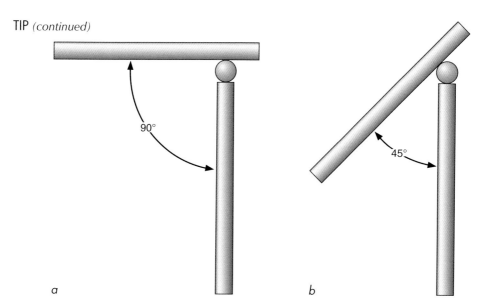

Figure 1.18 Illustration exaggerating a pelvis that is higher on one side than the other and the effect of this on the right hip.

Next, consider the ischium. In the illustration in figure 1.19, can you see that it is elevated on the right? What consequences might this have for the length of the hamstring muscles? If the knee joints were level, could the left hamstrings be shorter than those on the right? These findings are summarised in table 1.1.

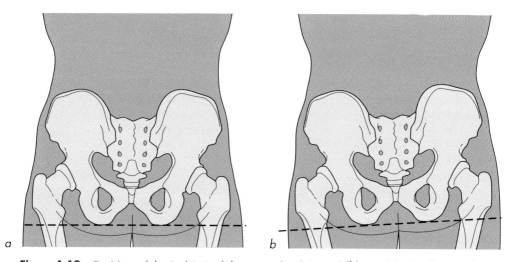

Figure 1.19 Position of the ischia in *(a)* a neutral pelvis and *(b)* a pelvis tilted upwards on the right.

Consequences
The consequences of a lateral pelvic tilt can be seen in table 1.1.

Posterior View

Posterior Superior Iliac Spines

The posterior superior iliac spines (PSIS) are located directly beneath the dimples some clients have in this region (figure 1.20a). In the photos in figures 1.20b and 1.20c, the position of the dimples suggests that the right PSIS is higher than the left PSIS in each example. Do you think the spine in each photo is straight or slightly flexed laterally to the right?

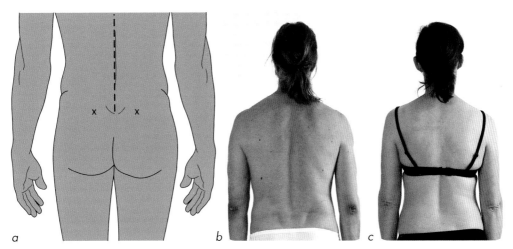

a   b   c

Figure 1.20 (a) Location of the PSIS. (b, c) Examples of clients whose right PSIS is higher than their left PSIS.

Photos b and c courtesy of Emma Kelly Photography.

TIP

Placing your thumbs over the PSIS dimples and observing your thumbs with respect to one another can help you gauge whether the PSIS points are level and therefore whether there may be any lateral pelvic tilt.

Consequences

If you determine that the left and right PSIS should be positioned on the same horizontal plane, yet you observe one to be higher, this suggests that the pelvis is laterally tilted. The consequences of a lateral pelvic tilt are shown in table 1.1.

Posterior View

Buttock Crease

It is not always possible or appropriate to observe the crease of the buttock where it meets the proximal thigh (see figure 1.21). If the client is wearing long shorts or cycling shorts, you will not be able to see these creases.

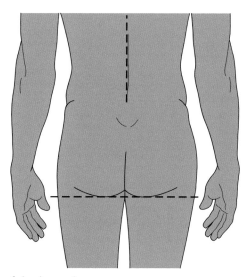

Figure 1.21   Location of the buttock crease.

TIP

The buttock crease is formed by the fat overlying the buttock muscles and does not indicate the location of the inferior fibres of the gluteus maximus muscle.

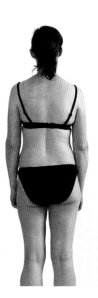

The person in figure 1.22 is a good example of someone with uneven buttock creases. Observe the position of their underwear too. Does it look like the right side of the pelvis is higher than the left? Could either the right tibia or femur, or both, be longer than the left, causing the pelvis to be raised on the right?

Figure 1.22   Example of uneven buttock creases.
Courtesy of Emma Kelly Photography.

Consequences

Clients who bear weight more on one side of the body than the other may have a deeper buttock crease on that side. This is also often true of clients with a laterally tilted pelvis. Thus, a client with a pelvis tilted upwards on the right (figure 1.22) might appear to have a deeper left buttock crease. Could differences in the depth of the buttock creases also correspond with leg-length discrepancies? Figure 1.23 illustrates the appearance of varying bone lengths in the lower limb with respect to the buttocks.

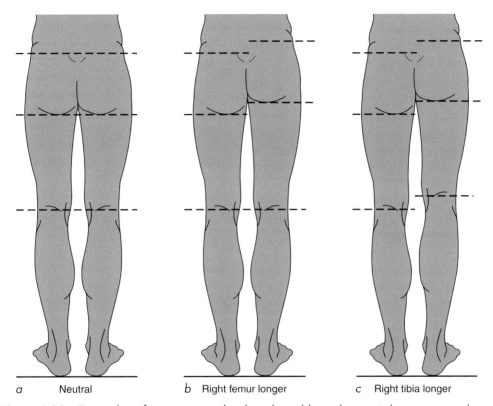

a   Neutral   b   Right femur longer   c   Right tibia longer

Figure 1.23 Examples of variations in leg length and how these might appear and affect the position of the buttock crease.

Posterior View

Pelvic Rotation

You learned that rotation of the pelvis can be assessed by comparing the position of the ASIS of your client in the anterior view. You can also assess for pelvic rotation in the posterior view, by observing the position of the PSIS. As with the anterior view, it helps to imagine your client is standing between two sheets of glass and to ask yourself which side of the pelvis would touch the glass if there were pelvic rotation. Which side of the pelvis would be closer to you? Figure 1.24 shows a neutral pelvis in the centre (1.24b) and provides exaggerated examples of rotation (1.24a and 1.24c).

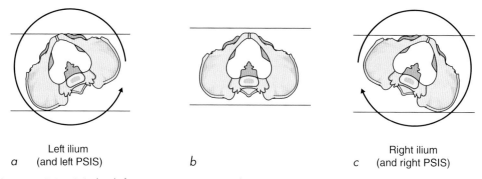

Left ilium		Right ilium
a (and left PSIS)	b	c (and right PSIS)

Figure 1.24 *(a)* The left posterior superior iliac spine (PSIS) is closer to the examiner. *(b)* Neutral pelvis. *(c)* The right PSIS is closer to the examiner.

TIP

Your findings in the posterior view should correspond with your findings in the anterior view. That is, if your client's left PSIS is closer to you in the posterior view, it must be farther away from you in the anterior view (figure 1.25).

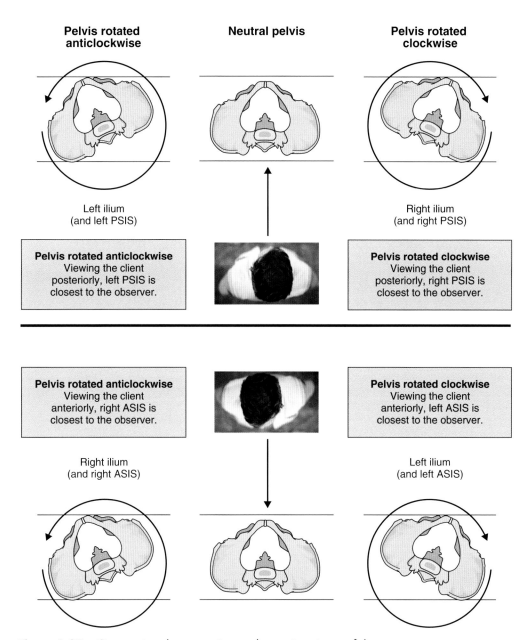

Figure 1.25 Comparing the posterior and anterior views of the same posture.

Consequences

The consequences of pelvic rotation are described in the corresponding section of the anterior postural assessment.

Posterior View

Internal Rotation of the Hip

As part of the anterior postural assessment, you looked to see whether there was any internal rotation of the lower limbs and learned that there may be internal or external rotation of an entire limb, or part of that limb. Internal rotation of the hip is internal rotation around the long axis of the femur. A patient with this posture may have a characteristic toe-in foot position, where the tibia is also internally rotated, or the foot position may be neutral. Unlike some of the other postures with signs that are visibly apparent, the degree of inward rotation of the femur is more difficult to identify from postural assessment alone, and for this reason, muscle length tests are important for determining whether a patient has a reduction in external hip rotation, which is a corresponding finding with this posture.

It is important to note that internal rotation of the hip is not the same as internal torsion of the femur. Femoral torsion is rotation *within* a bone itself, a twisting of the bone, whereas internal rotation of the hip occurs *between* bones, at the coxofemoral joint. Each results in a change in the orientation of the femoral condyles in the transverse plane. Thus, observing the client's knees anteriorly and posteriorly can be helpful in identifying internal rotation of the hip. With both internal rotation of the hip and internal femoral torsion, the lateral femoral condyle is orientated more anteriorly than typical, and the medial femoral condyle is orientated more posteriorly. In the patient shown in figure 1.26a, the lateral femoral condyle of the left femur is anteriorly orientated and disappears in a posterior view, whereas the medial femoral condyle is posteriorly orientated and appears more prominent. This indicates internal rotation of the left hip or internal femoral torsion on that side.

TIP

To help you identify internal rotation when viewing a client posteriorly, imagine the popliteal spaces as if they were the headlights on a car (see figure 1.26b), just as you did when observing the knees anteriorly. Kneeling squarely behind your client but about 2 metres (2.2 yd) from them, ask yourself where the headlight beams would fall. Would a beam be directed towards you (indicating neutral tibiofemoral alignment) or to one side (indicating hip rotation or femoral torsion)? Observe that the popliteal spaces on this patient's right and left knees are not orientated in the same direction; a beam from the left-knee headlight would fall to your left, whereas a beam from the right-knee headlight would fall closer to you.

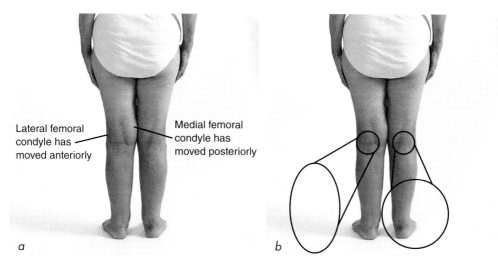

Lateral femoral condyle has moved anteriorly

Medial femoral condyle has moved posteriorly

a

b

Figure 1.26 *(a)* A patient with internal rotation of the left hip (internal femoral torsion). *(b)* Imagining the popliteal spaces as vehicle headlights.

Photos courtesy of Emma Kelly Photography.

It is tempting to conclude that a person standing with forward-facing feet does not have any internal rotation at the hip joint. Remember that in typical standing, the feet turn outwards slightly by about 6 to 8 degrees, so a patient with feet facing forwards could have an internally rotated hip, internal tibial torsion, internal femoral torsion or a combination. (A section on tibial torsion appeared earlier in this chapter.)

The subject of internal hip rotation can be confusing because both internal rotation of the femur and internal femoral torsion contribute to torsion of the entire lower limb. Inward rotation of the entire lower limb may be the result of a combination of factors at the coxofemoral and knee joints and within the femur and tibia. As with many of the postures described in this book, it is important to clarify the degree of internal rotation you suspect using muscle length tests rather than relying on postural assessment alone.

Consequences

With increased internal hip rotation, there is corresponding decreased external rotation in the coxofemoral joint. Internal rotators are shortened, and external rotators are lengthened (table 1.9). Both muscle groups may be weakened because they are not functioning at their optimal length or within their optimal range. Weakness in external rotators of the hip is associated with musculoskeletal disorders of the knee, such as patellofemoral joint pain syndrome and non-contact injury to the anterior cruciate ligament in adolescent girls (Neumann 2010). Imbalance in muscles around the hip joint could affect the function of the joint and ultimately could affect not only gait but also functional and sporting activities.

Femoral torsion can be a contributing factor to internal rotation of the hip. The degree of femoral torsion is described as an angle that is formed by a line drawn longitudinally through the neck of the femur, superimposed over a line drawn between the femoral condyles. This angle is usually 10 to 15 degrees but varies widely. An increase in torsion angle is called anteversion, which can cause compensatory change in the hip joint and affect weight bearing, muscle biomechanics and hip joint stability. It may also create dysfunction at the knee and foot (Levangie and Norkin 2001).

Internal rotation of the hip changes the neutral orientation of the femoral head within the acetabulum. Prolonged alteration in the distribution of forces through the articular surfaces of the hip joint could predispose the joint to degenerative changes in the bone, articular cartilage and connective tissue. Internal rotation of the hip threatens to pinch anterior hip structures, causing pain.

With internal rotation of the femur, there is atypical orientation of the knee joint. This is exacerbated where there is a neutral foot position, because this requires external rotation of the tibia in cases where internal rotation of the femur is present. Altered hip and knee biomechanics alter both walking and running ability and could therefore adversely affect participation in recreational and sporting activities. Where internal rotation is due to torsional deformity of the femur, this could contribute to arthritis in the knee joint: Internal femoral torsion increases pressure on the lateral facet, producing anterior knee pain and patellofemoral arthritis. There may be lateral patellar subluxation.

Internal rotation of the hip is often accompanied by subtalar pronation of the foot, and this also causes problems (more information is provided later in this chapter).

Table 1.9   Muscle Lengths Associated With Internal Rotation of the Hip

Area	Shortened muscles	Lengthened muscles
Hip	Tensor fasciae latae	Gluteus maximus
	Gluteus minimus	Gluteus medius (posterior fibres)
	Gluteus medius (anterior fibres)	Piriformis
	Adductor longus	Quadratus femoris
	Adductor brevis	Obturator
	Adductor magnus	Gemelli muscles
	Pectineus	Psoas
	Gracilis	Sartorius

TIP

Note that the piriformis, posterior fibres of the gluteus minimus and anterior fibres of the gluteus maximus change from being external to internal rotators as the hip is progressively flexed.

Posterior View

Muscle Bulk and Tone

As with the anterior assessment, compare the shape and size of the thighs and calves, asking yourself whether there is any hypertrophy or atrophy (figure 1.27).

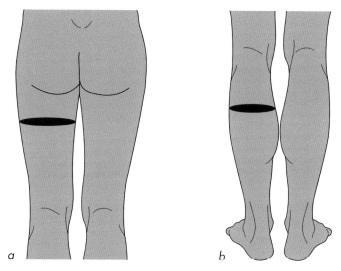

Figure 1.27 Checking the girth of the *(a)* thigh and *(b)* calf.

Consequences

Greater thigh or calf bulk on one side suggests an increased use of the thigh or calf muscles of that leg with respect to the other. An alternative explanation might be poor lymphatic drainage, as is seen in patients with lymphoedema; in this case, the limb will appear swollen rather than there being an increase in muscle bulk. Limb atrophy may be observed in clients after illness or immobility and is due to muscle atrophy.

TIP

Clients who have injured a leg, foot or ankle are often observed to have less bulk in the lower limb on that side, simply because they are using that limb less. This may be accompanied by a compensatory increase in the muscle bulk of the other side. For example, a client recovering from a ruptured right Achilles tendon, a fractured ankle or toe surgery could have reduced bulk on the right lower limb and increased bulk on the left lower limb. Injuries that occurred when your client was a child or teenager may manifest in asymmetry between the lower limbs, because reduced weight bearing during childhood may have affected muscle and bone development. Although it is subtle, you may observe some clients shifting their weight laterally, with a subconscious disinclination to bear weight on the side of a former injury.

Posterior View

Posterior Knee

Take a look at the posterior aspect of the knee and note anything unusual about it. Does your client stand with neutral, flexed or hyperextended knees? Although this is best assessed when you carry out the lateral postural assessment, you can sometimes get a feel for knee position by observing how prominent the popliteal area appears to be. Is there any oedema, or are there signs of bursitis? You learned in the anterior assessment to look for genu varum and valgum. Check for this also when carrying out your posterior assessment. Figure 1.28 is an example of someone with a slight genu valgum posture of the right knee.

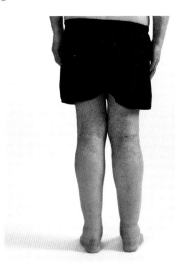

Figure 1.28 Slight genu valgum of the right knee.

Courtesy of Emma Kelly Photography.

Consequences

The consequences will depend on whether the client has a flexed or hyperextended knee. These postures are best determined in the lateral view, combined with range-of-motion tests.

TIP

If the posterior knee seems more deeply creased than typical, this could indicate that the client is standing with a flexed knee. If the posterior knee is prominent, with the popliteus muscle seeming to protrude slightly, this could indicate that the client is hyperextending at this joint. Bursitis presents with an obvious protrusion.

Posterior View

Calf Midline

Imagine a line running vertically down the centre of the client's calf from the knee crease through the Achilles tendon (figure 1.29). If necessary, draw this line using a body crayon. Compare the left and right calves and their relationship to the midline of the body. Look also at the shape of the legs and whether there is evidence of tibial bowing.

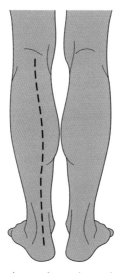

Figure 1.29   Use an imagined or drawn line along the midline of the calf.

TIP

One way to understand how hip rotation can affect the position of the calf is to draw the vertical calf lines on your client and then stand back and observe these lines when you instruct the client to alter their hip position. Ask them first to stand with one foot pigeon-toed. Compare the calf line on this leg with that of the other leg, and you will see that the line has moved outwards, away from the midline of the body, because the client has rotated the hip internally to stand pigeon-toed. Then ask the client to turn their foot out on that side whilst keeping the other foot facing forwards or in a neutral position. This time, the opposite happens: The calf line moves inwards, towards the midline of the body, as the client contracts the external hip rotators.

Consequences

The experiment described in the preceding tip box demonstrates that a line that appears to be lateral (rather than central) on the calf could result from an internally rotated hip on that side or a tibia that is medially rotated against the femur on that side. In either case, the foot position may also change when the person stands pigeon-toed. A line that appears to be medial (rather than central) on the calf indicates the opposite: an externally rotated hip on that side or a tibia that is laterally rotated against the femur on that side. In this case, the client may stand with the feet turned out. Table 1.10 summarises this information and provides a reminder of the muscles acting on the hip to bring about either internal or external rotation.

If a client comes to you with a hip problem, a postural assessment is a good place to start, because it may reveal shortness in one group of muscles and the need to test for tightness in these muscles later. Remember that it is ultimately important to discern whether the position of the calf is due to imbalances in hip muscles or torsion in the tibia, because your treatment protocol will be different for each.

Bowing of the tibia could indicate osteomalacia or increased compressive forces on the concave side of the bone.

Table 1.10 Calf Line and Corresponding Effects on the Feet and the Leg Muscles

	Calf line appears lateral	Calf line appears medial
Position of the hip, tibia or both	Indicates internal rotation of the hip, the tibia or both	Indicates external rotation of the hip, the tibia or both
Foot position	Sometimes, the client stands pigeon-toed	Sometimes, the client stands with the feet turned out
Muscles that may be shortened	Internal rotators of the hip: Gluteus minimus Gluteus medius (anterior fibres) Adductors Pectineus Gracilis	External rotators of the hip: Gluteus maximus Gluteus medius (posterior fibres) Piriformis Quadratus femoris Obturator Gemelli muscles Psoas* Sartorius

*The psoas is not a definitive rotator, yet it may be more involved in stability of the spine, including rotation, than originally thought.

Posterior View

Achilles Tendon

Observation of the ankles can provide clues relating to pain and dysfunction not only in the ankle itself but also in the feet and knees. Start by looking at the Achilles tendon and the position of the calcaneus. Figure 1.30 shows six ankles belonging to three clients. Observe the variety of shapes of the Achilles tendon, the position of the calcaneus and the position of the ankle joint itself, plus the foot position chosen by clients when undergoing postural assessment.

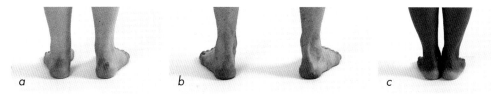

a   b   c

Figure 1.30   Observe the Achilles tendon.
Courtesy of Emma Kelly Photography.

It can be helpful to use a body crayon to draw a line vertically down the Achilles tendon, over the calcaneus and to the floor (figure 1.31), then to stand back and observe the line you have drawn. Is the tendon straight, concave or convex? Do the feet appear to roll out or to roll in? You can read more detailed information about ankle postures in the sections on pes valgus and pes varus.

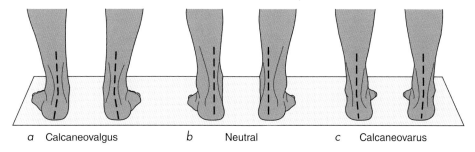

a   Calcaneovalgus   b   Neutral   c   Calcaneovarus

Figure 1.31   *(a)* Calcaneovalgus, *(b)* neutral and *(c)* calcaneovarus postures.

Consequences

The observation of the Achilles tendon can help provide information about excessive ankle eversion or inversion. Clients with excessive eversion, sometimes popularly referred to as overpronation, may have shortened peroneal (fibular) muscles on that leg.

Posterior View

Pes Valgus (Pronated Foot)

The positions of the malleoli provide clues as to whether your client has a neutral ankle position (figure 1.32a) or whether there is evidence of pes valgus (figure 1.32b) or pes varus. *Pes* is a term restricted to any foot deformity of acquired origin, and *valgus* refers to bones distal to the joint moving in a single plane away from the midline (Ritchie and Keim 1964). In the pes valgus foot posture (pronated foot), the calcaneus is the bone that moves away from the midline and is often described as being abducted (figure 1.32b). Another way to describe the pes valgus posture is that there is eversion (or valgus) of the heel. There is pronation of the foot, and the medial longitudinal arch is reduced in height.

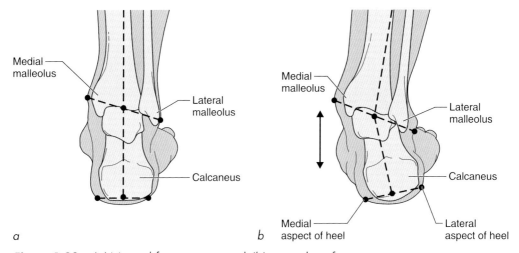

Figure 1.32 *(a)* Neutral foot posture and *(b)* pes valgus foot posture.

The posture is easy to identify because in neutral foot posture, the lateral malleolus is positioned slightly inferior to the medial malleolus, whereas in the pes valgus posture, the lateral malleolus lies even lower. Your client may appear to be bearing weight more on the medial side of the heel (often evidenced by increased wear on the sole of the shoe), with less pressure on the lateral side of the heel. When assessing a client, it can sometimes be helpful to imagine a line through the tibia, talus and calcaneus; in the neutral foot posture, it is vertical, but it deviates in the pes valgus posture, forming an obtuse angle on the lateral side of the ankle.

The person in figure 1.33 has prominent medial malleoli. Could it be that her tibiae are twisted so that each knee turns inwards as the whole of the tibia, including the distal end, rotates medially? Could that explain why we can see more of the medial malleoli on both the left and right ankles?

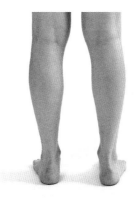

Figure 1.33 Observe the malleoli to help determine ankle posture.
Courtesy of Emma Kelly Photography.

Consequences

In the pes valgus posture, there are increased tensile stresses on the medial side of the ankle and increased compressive stresses on the lateral side of the ankle (figure 1.32*b*). Anatomic foot type does not appear to be a risk factor for ankle sprains (Beynnon, Murphy, and Alosa 2002), although many studies have tested participants standing barefoot and not dynamically. Nevertheless, theoretically, increased tensile stress on the medial side of the ankle could lengthen and weaken the medial collateral (deltoid) ligament, predisposing a patient to medial collateral ankle sprain.

Ligaments between the tibia and fibula contribute to the function of both superior and inferior tibiofibular joints (Levangie and Norkin 2001). Compressive stress on the lateral side of the ankle could therefore affect the proper functioning not only of the distal tibiofibular joint but also of the proximal tibiofibular joint.

A pronated foot increases the likelihood of having hallux valgus and overlapping toes (Hagedorn et al. 2013) as well as metatarsalgia, interdigital neuritis and plantar fasciitis (Fowler 2004).

Table 1.11 illustrates muscle length changes associated with the pes valgus posture. Such changes may explain why a pronated foot requires more muscle work for maintaining stance stability than does a supinated foot (Magee 2002) and why there may be myositis or tendinitis of the tibialis anterior and tibialis posterior (Fowler 2004). People with pronated feet are more likely to have Achilles tendinitis or tendinosis due to greater demands placed on the tendon when walking (American College of Foot and Ankle Surgeons 2023a). Spindles in ankle muscles are significant for the control of posture and balance whilst walking (Sorensen, Holland, and Patla 2002). Muscles listed in table 1.11 all cross the ankle joint, and changes to their length or health are therefore likely to affect balance too. This could be particularly significant for older adults.

Fowler (2004) suggests that excessive foot pronation is associated with calcaneal bursitis and may contribute to medial knee injury, patellofemoral syndrome, iliotibial band syndrome, shin splints, trochanteric bursitis, anterior shift of the pelvis and lumbar facet syndrome along with sacrococcygeal dysfunction in the spine.

Patients with osteoarthritis in the medial compartment of the knee have been found to have a more pronated foot compared to control individuals (Levinger et al. 2010) and to walk with greater rearfoot eversion (Levinger et al. 2012), as in the pes valgus posture. It is not clear whether pes valgus develops in response to medial-compartment knee osteoarthritis or whether the foot posture itself contributes to the development of this knee pathology. There may be pain in both the medial and lateral sides of the talocrural joint (Gross 1995).

Proper joint movement in the foot and ankle is essential for neutral gait, and atypical pronation results in the inability of the foot to absorb the forces of weight bearing effectively (Donatelli 1987). In the pes valgus posture, the heel abducts (everts). In the closed chain (weight bearing), this forces the talus to adduct and leads to plantar flexion. The tibia follows the motion of the talus and thus is forced into slight internal rotation. Additionally, there may be internal rotation of the femur and rotation of the pelvis (Riegger-Krugh and Keysor 1996). Pes valgus may be associated with the genu valgum (knock-kneed) posture. Raising the lateral side of the foot (as in the pes valgus foot posture) results in significant changes in pelvic tilt and torsion (Betsch et al. 2011).

Given the changes in other joints of the lower limb associated with the pes valgus posture, it is easy to see why it is popularly believed that pes valgus may be associated with an increased risk of injury. However, measurements of static lower limb biomechanical alignment have not been found to be related to injury in recreational athletes (Lun et al. 2004).

Table 1.11 Muscle Lengths Associated With Pes Valgus

Area	Shortened muscles	Lengthened muscles
Ankle and leg	Fibular (peroneal) muscles Gastrocnemius Soleus	Tibialis posterior Adductor hallucis Flexor hallucis longus Flexor digitorum longus
Thigh	Where there are associated changes at the hip and knee: biceps femoris, hip adductors, tensor fasciae latae	Where there are associated changes at the hip and knee: gluteus maximus, gluteus medius

TIP

In addition to shortening of muscles on the lateral side of the leg, there may be tightness in the iliotibial band.

Posterior View

Pes Varus (Supinated Foot)

Just as with the pes valgus posture, you can use the position of the malleoli to determine whether your client has a neutral (figure 1.34a) or pes varus (figure 1.34b) ankle posture. The term *varus* means that bones distal to the joint move in a single plane towards the midline (Ritchie and Keim 1964). In the pes varus foot posture (supinated foot), the calcaneus is the bone that moves towards the midline, and it is often described as being adducted. Another way to describe the pes varus posture is to say that there is inversion (or varus) of the heel. There is supination of the foot, and the medial longitudinal arch may be accentuated.

In neutral foot posture, the lateral malleolus is positioned slightly inferior to the medial malleolus (figure 1.34a), whereas in the pes varus posture, the lateral malleolus lies higher, more parallel with the medial malleolus (figure 1.34b). Your client may appear to be bearing weight more on the lateral side of the heel, often evidenced by increased wear on the sole of the shoe, with less pressure on the medial side of the heel. When assessing a client, it can sometimes be helpful to imagine a line through the tibia, talus and calcaneus, which in the neutral foot posture is vertical but deviates in the pes varus posture, forming an obtuse angle on the medial side of the ankle.

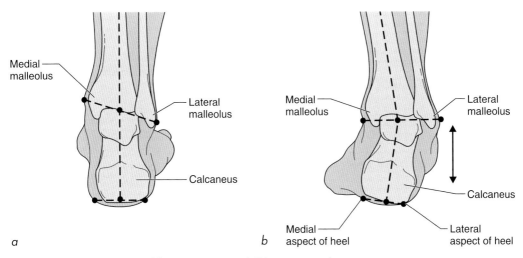

Figure 1.34 *(a)* Neutral foot posture and *(b)* pes varus foot posture.

Consequences

There are increased compressive stresses on the medial side of the ankle and increased tensile stresses on the lateral side of the ankle. It is commonly believed that the pes varus posture predisposes a patient to ankle sprains, and this could be due to weakening of the lateral collateral ankle ligaments as a result of increased tensile stress. However, as previously indicated, Beynnon, Murphy and Alosa (2002) reported that anatomic foot type does not appear to be a risk factor for ankle sprains.

Increased tensile stress on the lateral side of the ankle could affect the proper functioning of the distal tibiofibular joint. Because both the distal and superior tibiofibular joints are linked, ligaments between the tibia and fibula contribute to the function of both joints (Levangie and Norkin 2001).

Table 1.12 illustrates muscle length changes associated with the pes varus posture. Spindles in ankle muscles are significant for the control of posture and balance whilst walking (Sorensen, Holland, and Patla 2002). Muscles listed in table 1.12 all cross the ankle joint; changes to their length or health are therefore likely to affect balance. This could be particularly significant for older adults. Furthermore, in the pes varus posture, the toes are lifted from the ground, and often, there is flexion of the big toe as it attempts to regain contact with the ground. It is essential that the toes function properly, not just for balance but so that body weight can be distributed more evenly when standing and walking (Hughes, Clark, and Klenerman 1990).

In the pes varus posture, the heel adducts (inverts). In the closed chain (weight bearing), this forces the talus to abduct and dorsiflex. Because the tibia follows the motion of the talus, the tibia is thus forced to externally rotate. This posture is also associated with external rotation of the femur and rotation of the pelvis (Riegger-Krugh and Keysor 1996). The consequences of this can be found in the section on tibial torsion.

Patients with excessive supination may develop plantar fasciitis, heel spurs, Achilles tendinitis, metatarsalgia and calcaneal bursitis (Donatelli 1987).

As with pes valgus, changes in joints of the lower limb associated with pes varus contribute to the popular belief that this posture may be associated with an increased risk of injury. Measurements of static lower limb biomechanical alignment have not been found to be related to injury in recreational athletes (Lun et al. 2004). However, reviewing the research into predictive factors for lateral ankle sprains, Beynnon, Murphy and Alosa (2002) reported that increased hindfoot inversion (as is the case with an inverted heel) is a risk factor predisposing military trainees to lower extremity overuse injury.

Table 1.12 Muscle Lengths Associated With Pes Varus

Area	Shortened muscles	Lengthened muscles
Foot	Flexor hallucis longus Flexor digitorum longus Tibialis anterior	Fibular (peroneal) muscles Extensor digitorum longus Extensor hallucis longus

TIP

The plantar fascia on the sole of the foot is shortened.

Posterior View

Foot Position

You began the anterior postural assessment by observing the stance adopted by your client. Another useful factor to consider is the specific position of the feet. Each foot usually turns out equidistant from the midline of the body, but sometimes, a person favours a toe-in or toe-out position of one or both feet. Can you see how the client in figure 1.35 is standing with their right foot turned out slightly compared to their left?

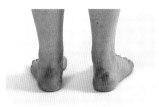

Figure 1.35 Example of external rotation of the right lower limb.
Courtesy of Emma Kelly Photography.

TIP

One way to assess foot position in the posterior view is to ask yourself how much of the lateral side of the foot you can see (i.e., how many toes). The more of the lateral aspect of the foot you can see (i.e., the more toes), the greater the degree of the toe-out position on that side.

Consequences

As you learned in the section on anterior assessment, the position of the foot (and leg) ties in with the position of the hip and tibia. Table 1.13 shows changes associated with toe-out and toe-in foot positions.

Table 1.13 Changes Associated With Toe-Out and Toe-In Foot Positions

	Toe-out position	Toe-in position
Possible position of the hip joint	Externally rotated	Internally rotated
Possible position of the tibia	Lateral tibial torsion	Medial tibial torsion
Muscles that might be shortened	External rotators of the femur; iliotibial band	Internal rotators of the femur

TIP

If, based on the position of the feet, you suspect that your client has shortened hip rotators, a crude but effective test is simply to ask them to stand in the foot position that would stretch those rotators. For example, if the client stands pigeon-toed, ask them to stand with the feet turned out like a ballet dancer. If the internal rotators really are tight, the client will find this toe-out position slightly uncomfortable.

Posterior View

Other Observations

Finally, as you did for the lower body anterior postural assessment, make note of any scars, blemishes or unusual marks on the client's skin. Has any strapping or taping been applied, perhaps in the treatment of an injury?

Lateral View

Overall Lower Limb Posture

Stand back and take an overall view of your client. Use of a plumb line can be helpful in assessing where ground forces may be affecting the lower limbs. The plumb line is positioned just anterior to the lateral malleolus (as shown in figure 1.36), and in a neutral posture, it bisects the leg, knee and pelvis. What do you notice about the lower limb postures of the clients in figure 1.37? Comparing each photograph to figure 1.36 reveals that none of these people have a neutral lower limb posture, because the plumb line does not bisect the legs, knees and pelvis equally. In addition, as might be expected, each of their postures differ. You will learn more about what the lateral assessment can reveal about the position of the pelvis, knees and ankles in later sections.

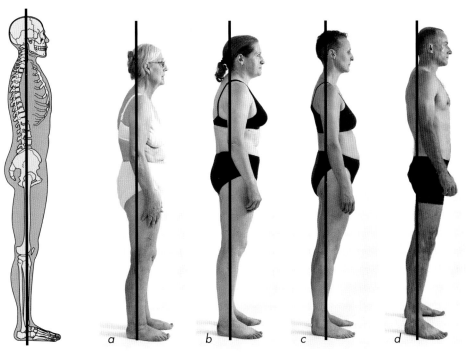

Figure 1.36   A plumb line drawn over a neutral posture.

Figure 1.37   Superimposing a plumb line over postural photographs.

Photos courtesy of Emma Kelly Photography.

TIP

With practice, you will learn to visualise a plumb line. If you are new to postural assessment, you may find it helpful to manually draw a plumb line over a photograph of your client or superimpose the line on a digital photograph.

Lateral View

Anterior Pelvic Tilt

When we walk, the pelvis naturally moves anteriorly and posteriorly (figure 1.38). *Anterior pelvic tilt* describes the position of the pelvis with the ASIS positioned anterior to the pubis in the sagittal plane.

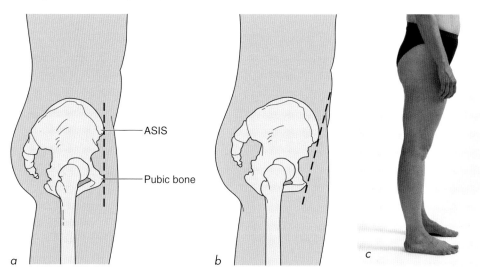

ASIS

Pubic bone

a *b* *c*

Figure 1.38 *(a)* A neutral pelvis. *(b)* An anteriorly tilted pelvis. *(c)* A client with an anteriorly tilted pelvis and the characteristic sloped appearance of the underwear.

Photo c courtesy of Emma Kelly Photography.

TIP

To better understand anterior and posterior pelvic tilting, try this: Standing, push your abdomen forwards and your buttocks out, extending your lumbar region. This produces an anterior pelvic tilt. Return to your neutral, resting position. Now contract your buttocks, pushing your groin forwards and flattening your lumbar spine. This produces a posterior pelvic tilt.

TIP

There is a trick to help you determine whether your client is standing with a particularly lordotic lumbar region or whether this region is flattened. Ask your client to perform the tilting manoeuvres you tried for yourself in the preceding tip. Once the client understands what to do, observe what occurs as they perform an anterior tilt and then a posterior tilt. If the client has difficulty tilting the pelvis anteriorly, increasing the lumbar curve, this could be because they are already in an anteriorly tilted position. If they have difficulty posteriorly tilting the pelvis, flattening the lumbar curve, this could be because they are already in a posteriorly tilted position.

Consequences

The position of the sacrum is associated with various degrees of spinal curvature, as is the shape of the auricular facet of the sacroiliac joint (SIJ) (Kapandji 2008). Compared with the position of the sacrum associated with a more neutral spine shape, in which there is increased curvature (and associated anterior pelvic tilt), the position of the sacrum becomes more horizontally orientated. This in itself may be of little consequence. However, the shape of the auricular facet has been found to vary amongst sacra associated with different spinal shapes, and it seems reasonable to assume that the shape of this facet suits the particular spinal shape with which it is associated. Could changing the orientation of the pelvis (and sacrum) from a neutral position to an anterior pelvic tilt have a detrimental effect on SIJ function by reducing the ability of this joint to withstand forces?

Nutation and counternutation are movements of the sacrum about an axis with respect to the ilia. (There is debate about where the axis of rotation lies.) With anterior pelvic tilt (red arrows in figure 1.39a), the sacrum moves in the opposite direction (blue arrows in figure 1.39a), a movement that has been termed *counternutation*. Looking at figure 1.39, consider the position in which the spine would move if there were no counternutation of the sacrum: Fixed at its base to the first sacral bone, the lumbar spine (and all of the vertebrae above it) would be forced forward, away from the vertical position. Counternutation is important because it marginally decreases the degree to which the spine must right itself back to vertical.

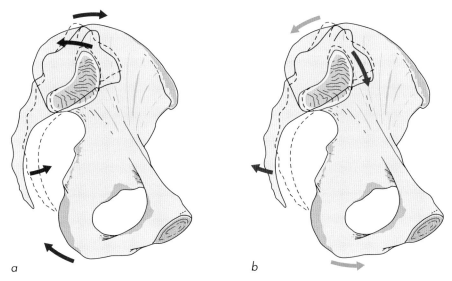

Figure 1.39 *(a)* Counternutation and *(b)* nutation of the sacrum, as seen in the anterior and posterior pelvic tilt conditions, respectively.

ANTERIOR PELVIC TILT

Where anterior pelvic tilt is pronounced or prolonged, could the sacrum be forced into counternutation for the spine to remain in a vertical position? What consequence might this have for the SIJ? Although the degree of SIJ movement is considered small (1-3 mm [0.0-0.1 in.]) (Houglum and Bertoti 2012), many therapists attribute back pain to dysfunction in this joint. Also, the sacral ligaments are strong and counter both nutation and counternutation. However, could prolonged anterior rotation of the pelvis stress the ligaments responsible for checking such movement, perhaps even affecting muscles associated with these ligaments (e.g., the superior tendon of the biceps femoris and the sacrotuberous ligament)?

Anterior movement of the acetabulum over the head of the femur changes the point of contact between these bony surfaces, the consequences of which are not known. Additionally, increased hip flexion corresponds with increased torque of the medial rotators of the hip and decreased torque of the lateral rotators. This could also affect the position of the femoral head in the acetabulum and the area of the head of the femur and acetabulum through which weight bearing and ground reaction forces are transmitted. Theoretically, this could lead to degenerative changes and adversely affect hip function in the long term.

An anteriorly tilted posture corresponds with an imbalance in flexor and extensor muscles (see the following list of factors corresponding to anterior pelvic tilt), which could adversely affect hip function. In addition, this posture corresponds with an increase in the lumbar curve and shares the consequences of that posture: As the pelvis tilts anteriorly, soft tissues of the posterior lumbar spine are compressed and greater pressure is placed on the posterior aspect of intervertebral discs than on the anterior lumbar spine, affecting nutrient exchange (Adams and Hutton 1985); facet joints are subject to increased stress, and there is a possibility of capsular strain (Scannell and McGill 2003). Imbalance between longitudinal ligaments of the lumbar spine could alter their stabilising capabilities; an anteriorly tilted pelvis could predispose a patient to osteoarthritis in lumbar facet joints, degenerative changes in parts of the lumbar discs and low back pain, and it could also give rise to symptoms affecting the lower limbs.

Factors Corresponding to Anterior Pelvic Tilt

Position of the ASIS: held anterior to the pubis

Corresponding position of the lumbar spine: increased lordosis

Shortened muscles: extensors of the lumbar spine, psoas major, rectus femoris, iliacus, tensor fasciae latae, sartorius

Lengthened muscles: rectus abdominis, hip extensors

Lateral View

Posterior Pelvic Tilt

Compared with a neutral pelvic posture (figure 1.40a), in the posterior pelvic tilt posture, the position of the ASIS is posterior to the pubis in the sagittal plane (figure 1.40b). With the lower limb fixed, posterior tilt of the pelvis produces hip extension and corresponds with a decrease in the lumbar curve. There is sometimes tension in the abdominal muscles, which may be observed by an increased transverse abdominal crease (figure 1.40c). As with anterior pelvic tilt, there is asymmetry in muscles of the anterior and posterior body (see the section on factors corresponding to posterior pelvic tilt).

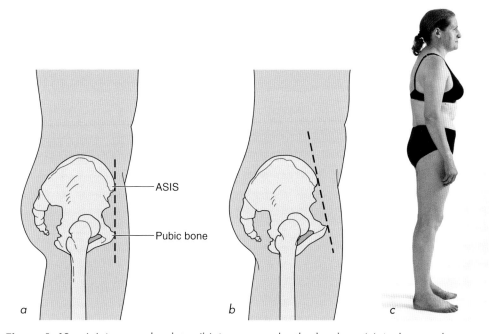

ASIS

Pubic bone

a   b   c

Figure 1.40 (a) A neutral pelvis. (b) A posteriorly tilted pelvis. (c) A client with a posteriorly tilted pelvis and an increased transverse abdominal crease.

Photo c courtesy of Emma Kelly Photography.

TIP

If there is tension in the abdominal muscles, they can pull on the anterior fascia, depressing the rib cage and hampering thoracic extension.

Consequences

Compared to a neutral pelvis, as the pelvis tilts posteriorly, the sacrum becomes more vertical and the coccygeal bones fall closer to vertical. Unless there is a significant change in pelvic tilt when seated, a patient with a posteriorly tilted pelvis could have coccygeal pain when sitting for prolonged periods.

With posterior tilt of the pelvis, the sacrum is forced into nutation (see figure 1.39*b*) for the spine to remain in a vertical position. As with the opposite posture (anterior pelvic tilt), changing the position of the SIJ, as well as the way it transmits forces from the ground and lower limbs to the spine and from the torso and upper limbs to the legs, could be detrimental to the functioning of this joint.

Factors corresponding to posterior pelvic tilt are listed here. As with hypolordosis of the lumbar spine, there is increased compressive stress on the anterior annuli of the discs and increased hydrostatic pressure in the nucleus at low load levels (Adams and Hutton 1985).

Factors Corresponding to Posterior Pelvic Tilt

Position of the ASIS: held posterior to the pubis

Corresponding position of the lumbar spine: decreased lordosis

Shortened muscles: lower abdominals, gluteus maximus

Lengthened muscles: lumbar erector spinae, psoas, iliacus, rectus femoris

Lateral View

Genu Recurvatum (Knee Hyperextension)

The lateral assessment is an excellent opportunity to observe what is happening at your client's knee joint. Commonly termed *knee hyperextension*, this posture describes extension at the knee (tibiofemoral) joint greater than neutral or zero degrees when weight bearing. Remember that when using a plumb line, you position your line just anterior to the lateral malleolus. This line bisects the tibia longitudinally in neutral knee posture (figure 1.41*a*). In the genu recurvatum posture, a larger portion of the calf falls posterior to the plumb line, which no longer bisects the leg (figure 1.41*b*). In this posture, the calf appears prominent in the lateral view, and the popliteal space appears prominent when you view your client posteriorly. The patella also appears to point downwards and to be compressed when you view your client anteriorly. The client shown in figure 1.41*c* is a good example of someone who stands with increased extension at the knee joint. Observe the front of this woman's knee. Can you see how it appears to be compressed, with the patella pushed into the front of the joint? Can you see how if you were to draw a plumb line onto this image, the leg would fall posterior to the plumb line? This posture is associated with excessive femoral internal rotation, genu varum or genu valgum, tibial varum and excessive subtalar joint pronation, all more apparent when you view your client anteriorly.

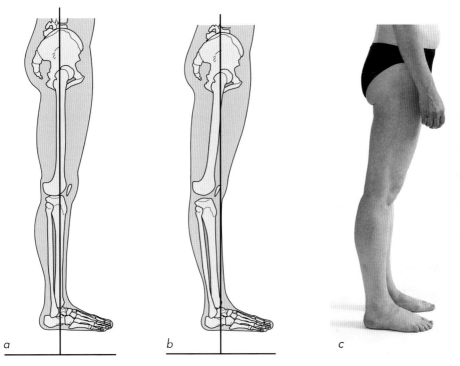

a *b* *c*

Figure 1.41 *(a)* Neutral knee alignment. *(b)* Genu recurvatum. *(c)* Mild genu recurvatum.

Photo *c* courtesy of Emma Kelly Photography.

TIP

If you can see more of the popliteal area (and perhaps also the calf) of the right leg when viewing the left side of the client, this indicates that the right knee is hyperextended. Being able to see more of the left leg when viewing the client's right side suggests that there may be increased extension in the left knee joint.

Consequences

In this posture, there is tension in posterior knee structures (such as the popliteus) and compression of anterior structures (such as the patellofemoral joint). As a consequence, adults who stand in knee hyperextension may have pain in the popliteal space (Kendall, McCreary, and Provance 1993) and patellofemoral pain. People with hypermobility have laxity in knee ligaments and stand in the genu recurvatum posture. The knee is the most painful joint in people with knee hypermobility, and patellofemoral pain syndrome is a common problem (Tinkle 2008).

Additionally, the typical kinematics of the knee are affected by alteration of tibiofemoral mechanics. In usual weight bearing, the femur rolls anteriorly and glides posteriorly on the fixed tibia, but in knee hyperextension, the femur tilts forwards, resulting in anterior compression of the femur and tibia. In weight bearing, capsular and ligamentous structures of the posterior knee are at risk of injury, and this in turn may lead to functional gait deficits. Patients with genu recurvatum posture walk more slowly than is typical, and many have higher knee extensor torque values than people with neutral knee posture (Kerrigan, Deming, and Holden 1996).

Other joints are also affected. There is increased hip extension and decreased ankle dorsiflexion, both of which are likely to affect gait and impair sporting performance that relies on lower limb agility. At the hip, there can be excessive anterior tilt. The genu recurvatum posture results in gait deviation and requires greater effort to maintain forward momentum (Fish and Kosta 1998).

The quadriceps and soleus muscles are shortened, and the knee extensor muscles are lengthened. Imbalance between knee flexors and extensors compromises the function and stability of both the knee and hip joints. Stretching of the popliteus reduces its ability to rotate the leg medially on the thigh and flex the knee and therefore affects optimal knee function. There may be a proprioceptive deficit near the end of the range of extension (Loudon, Goist, and Loudon 1998), and patients may feel the sensation of knee instability.

A positive correlation between genu recurvatum and anterior cruciate ligament injury in female athletes has been found (Loudon, Goist, and Loudon 1998). Genu recurvatum posture may predispose female athletes to overuse injuries of the knee (Devan et al. 2004). Knee hyperextension may be prevalent in some swimmers, and it has been postulated that this is the result of overstretching of the cruciate ligaments due to repetitive kicking. This posture gives a greater range of anterior-to-posterior motion at the knee, but it is not clear whether genu recurvatum is advantageous to swimmers (Bloomfield, Ackland, and Elliott 1994).

Factors corresponding to the genu recurvatum posture are listed here.

Factors Corresponding to Genu Recurvatum

Shortened muscles: quadriceps, soleus

Lengthened muscles: gastrocnemius

Hip position: increased hip extension

Ankle position: decreased dorsiflexion

Other: stretching of the posterior joint capsule of the knee; increased likelihood of degenerative changes to the patellofemoral joint

Lateral View

Genu Flexum (Flexed Knee)

As the name indicates, in the genu flexum (flexed knee) posture, a person bears weight through a knee that is flexed to a greater degree than is typical when standing. Less common than genu recurvatum, this posture is observed in older patients or in patients who have been sedentary and whose knees have been allowed to rest in a flexed position for prolonged periods. Viewed laterally, an imaginary line drawn vertically from just anterior to the lateral malleolus bisects the tibia longitudinally in neutral knee posture (figure 1.42a). In the genu flexum posture, the knee itself falls anterior to this line, which no longer bisects the leg (figure 1.42b). This posture is best identified by viewing your client in the sagittal plane, as with the patient in figure 1.42c. Note the increased ankle dorsiflexion commonly associated with this posture.

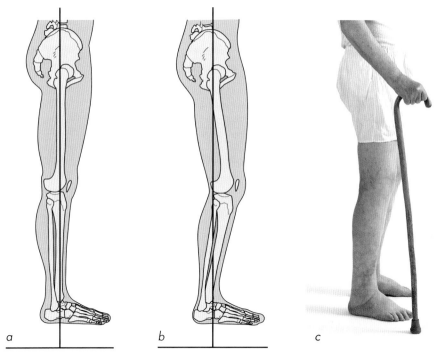

a   b   c

Figure 1.42 *(a)* Neutral knee alignment. *(b)* Genu flexum. *(c)* A client with genu flexum of the right leg.

Photo c courtesy of Emma Kelly Photography.

Consequences

When the knee is extended, the collateral ligaments are relatively taut, helping to stabilise the joint. They slacken when the knee flexes and permit some axial rotation. Repeated weight bearing through a flexed knee could increase the likelihood of rotational injury to the knee.

Constant muscular effort is required for standing in knee flexion, which can be fatiguing. Constant contraction of the quadriceps has another disadvantage. This muscle exerts a pull on the tibia at the insertion of the tibial tuberosity, and this could lead to tenderness or the development of unwanted teno-osseous pathology. There is increased pressure on the anterior aspect of the ankle due to increased dorsiflexion.

Prolonged unilateral knee flexion is associated with pronation of the foot and medial rotation of the contralateral thigh along with ipsilateral hip drop (contralateral hip hitch), convex curving of the spine towards the affected side and contralateral drop of the shoulder (Kendall, McCreary, and Provance 1993). For example, a patient with right knee flexion is more likely to have pronation of the left foot, internal rotation of the left thigh, a dropped hip on the right side (but a raised hip on the left side) and a dropped left shoulder.

Factors corresponding to the genu flexum posture are listed here.

Factors Corresponding to Genu Flexum

Shortened muscles: hamstrings, popliteus

Lengthened muscles: quadriceps, soleus

Hip position: increased hip flexion

Ankle position: increased dorsiflexion

Other: increased pressure on structures of the anterior ankle joint

TIP

Swelling of the knee can make it difficult to determine if someone has a genu flexum knee posture. This is a good example of why additional tests should always be used when assessing a joint. In this example, the additional tests would include active and passive knee flexion and extension.

Lateral View

Ankle Position

Examine your client's ankles. Are they neutral, or do you notice any increased or decreased dorsiflexion? Decreased dorsiflexion is associated with the genu recurvatum posture, whereas increased dorsiflexion is associated with genu flexum. The three people in figure 1.43 are good examples of individuals with decreased dorsiflexion at the ankle, as is common with knee hyperextension.

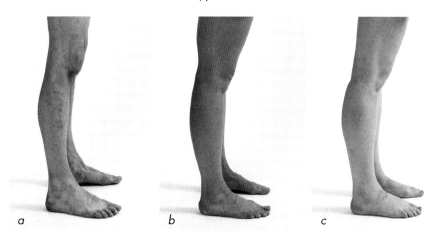

a   b   c

Figure 1.43 Examples of decreased ankle dorsiflexion.

Courtesy of Emma Kelly Photography.

Consequences

Increased dorsiflexion in standing is observed in clients who stand with flexed knees. In these clients, ground forces are no longer distributed evenly up through the tibiae during walking. Possible consequences might be pain and early degenerative joint changes. There may be a shortened tibialis anterior muscle and increased pressure to the anterior aspect of the ankle retinaculum. Decreased dorsiflexion is associated with shortened quadriceps and increased pressure to the anterior of the knee joint.

TIP

As when observing genu recurvatum, ankle position can be masked by swelling. Here again, it is advisable to perform range-of-motion tests in addition to your postural assessment to determine whether there are any restrictions in the joint, or conversely, whether there is increased laxity.

Lateral View

Pes Cavus (High Arches)

You have probably heard people speak about having 'flat feet' or 'high arches'. These are lay terms for positions of the foot bones. Observing whether your client has an exaggerated foot posture is helpful in determining the kinds of forces that might be passing through their lower limbs. In the pes cavus posture (high arches), the calcaneus is supinated, and the plantar arch is higher (figure 1.44c) compared to a neutral foot (figure 1.44a). There is a greater-than-usual space between the floor and the medial side of the foot. Typically, there is a varus (inverted) hindfoot, a plantar flexed first metatarsal, an adducted forefoot and claw toes (Burns et al. 2007). Footprints of a patient with pes cavus reveal reduced contact points with the ground (figure 1.44d) compared to footprints of a patient with a neutral foot posture (figure 1.44b). In observing this posture, look for claw toes, splaying of the forefoot and a raised arch. Posteriorly, you may observe that the calcaneus is supinated (pes varus).

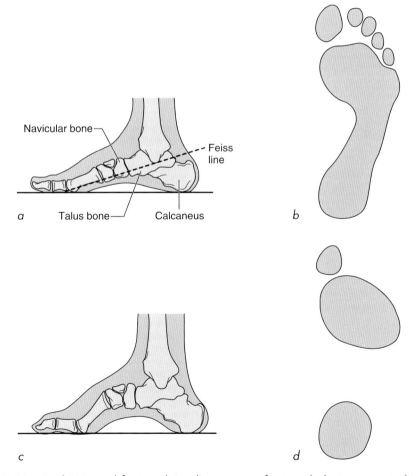

a   Navicular bone — Feiss line — Talus bone — Calcaneus   b

c   d

Figure 1.44 *(a, b)* Neutral foot and *(c, d)* pes cavus foot, with their associated footprints.

TIP

Many providers of sport footwear now have pressure plates on-site to assess how potential buyers distribute their weight both when standing and running. A crude way to determine weight bearing when standing is simply to take footprints. This is not something that is usually done as part of a postural assessment, but it is a fun activity to carry out at home to clarify your observations of family and friends.

Consequences

In the pes cavus posture, there is increased pressure on the ball of the foot. It is suggested that patients with pes cavus may have hammertoes or claw toes; calluses on the ball, side or heel of the foot; pain when standing or walking; and an increased likelihood of ankle sprains due to the heel tilting inwards (supinating) (American College of Foot and Ankle Surgeons 2023b).

Individuals with pes cavus sometimes have difficulty finding footwear that fits and have reduced tolerance for walking (Burns et al. 2007). Runners with high arches report a greater incidence of ankle injuries, bony injuries and lateral injuries (Williams, McClay, and Hamill 2001). There may be painful calluses beneath the metatarsal heads, caused by loss of the metatarsal arch, and there also may be osteoarthritic changes in the tarsal region (Magee 2002).

If the subtalar and transverse tarsal joints are locked into supination, this will prevent shock absorption, and the hindfoot supination may cause rotational stress on the leg (Levangie and Norkin 2001). As with pes planus, an alteration in foot function affects the entire kinetic chain of the lower limb.

Anatomical and functional changes associated with the pes cavus posture are listed here.

Changes Associated With Pes Cavus

Change in plantar arch: higher than typical

Change in the position of the foot bones: the calcaneus supinates; the remainder of the foot pronates

Change in soft tissues: shortening of the intrinsic foot muscles and the plantar fascia; where there are claw toes, the associated toe extensor tendons are short

Relationship to trunk rotation: trunk rotation to the left increases supination of the left foot and pressure through the lateral side of the left foot; trunk rotation to the right increases supination of the right foot and pressure through the lateral side of the right foot

TIP

With the longitudinal arch raised, the opposite ends of the arch are brought closer together, and there is shortening of the plantar fascia.

Lateral View

Pes Planus (Flatfoot)

Commonly termed *flatfoot*, pes planus differs from the neutral foot posture (figure 1.45a), and the footprint of a person with pes planus differs from the footprint a neutral foot produces (figure 1.45b). In the pes planus foot posture, there is loss of the typical longitudinal plantar arch, giving the foot a flattened appearance (figure 1.45c). When pes planus is present in both weight-bearing and non–weight-bearing positions, it is known as *rigid flatfoot*. When the arch is absent in standing but present in non–weight-bearing positions, it is termed *flexible flatfoot*. In this posture, there is excessive pronation as the talus glides medially over the calcaneus and comes into contact with the ground. The medial side of the foot may be touching the floor completely, leaving no gap at all. This is reflected by the shape of the footprint (figure 1.45d), which shows greater surface area than usual because a greater portion of the sole is in contact with the ground. The flattened appearance of the foot makes this an easy posture to identify in a patient (figure 1.45e).

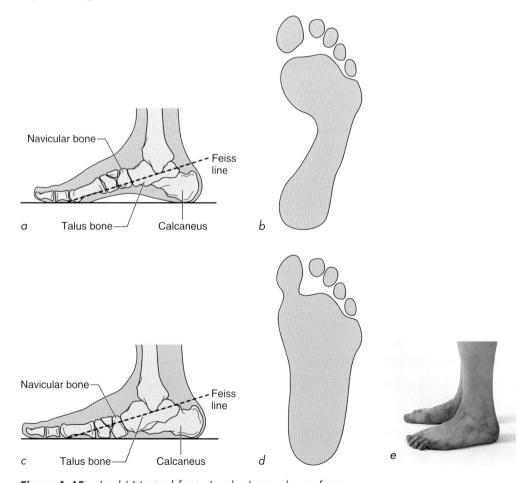

Figure 1.45 *(a, b)* Neutral foot; *(c, d, e)* pes planus foot.
Photo *e* courtesy of Emma Kelly Photography.

Pes planus occurs when the navicular bone (figure 1.45c) lies beneath the Feiss line, a line running from the top of the medial malleolus to the base of the first metatarsal in the neutral foot (figure 1.45a).

In addition to flattening of the foot, when you observe the client from behind, you may notice that the toes drift outwards and the ankle appears to fall inwards as the calcaneus pronates (the pes valgus ankle posture). Pes planus is considered mild if hindfoot valgus is 4 to 6 degrees, moderate if it is 6 to 10 degrees, and severe if it is 10 to 15 degrees (Magee 2002). For more information on calcaneal pronation, see the section on the pes valgus posture.

Consequences

The arch of the foot provides a spring mechanism essential for helping to absorb and dissipate forces during gait. Loss of the arch means reduced shock absorption, which could contribute to the development of stress injuries to the feet, the ankles and the bones of the legs. In some cases, the pes planus posture could impair balance and stability. However, studies carried out using military personnel did not support the notion of increased incidence of injury in patients with flat feet (Giladi et al. 1987; Jones et al. 1993).

During the midstance of gait, the foot pronates slightly via the talus and goes into slight supination during push-off. The tibia responds to these movements by rotating internally and then externally. Therefore, a talus that is incorrectly placed or does not function optimally hinders tibial function and affects the entire kinetic chain of the lower limb. The gait of a patient with pes planus has been described as slouchy and jarring, with exaggerated flexion of the knee and weight bearing on the heel, such that the demands of muscular activity are increased (Whitman 2010). An increase in tension in the muscles of the feet whilst walking has been found in patients with pes planus, which could explain why people with flat feet experience pain when they walk for long periods (Fan et al. 2011).

People with flexible flatfoot are more likely to have hammertoes and overlapping toes (Hagedorn et al. 2013). These can cause discomfort and difficulty wearing certain types of footwear.

Individuals with severe pes planus have pain. In addition to pain in the heel, arch and ankle and along the outside of the foot, there may be pain in the shinbone and even low back, hip or knee (American College of Foot and Ankle Surgeons 2023b). There may be pain and swelling of the tibialis posterior tendon and pain not only during activities such as running but also when walking or standing (American Academy of Orthopedic Surgeons 2023).

The pes planus foot posture stretches and weakens the plantar aponeurosis and the intrinsic muscles of the foot and ligaments. Patients with hypermobility syndromes who already have increased laxity in the ligaments of the foot may have pain and weakness in the foot, ankle and leg (Tinkle 2008).

Specimens of the tibialis posterior tendon taken from patients with adult-acquired flatfoot reveal the presence of enzymes that break down and weaken the tendon (Corps et al. 2012).

Dysfunction of the posterior tibial tendon results in relative internal rotation of the tibia and talus and a flattening of the medial arch. Over time, this contributes to deformity of the ankle, eventually leading the calcaneus to impinge against the fibula, causing pain (Myerson 1996).

Anatomical and functional changes associated with the pes planus posture are listed here.

Changes Associated With Pes Planus

Change in plantar arch: loss of the plantar arch

Change in the position of the foot bones: the talus glides medially over the calcaneus

Change in soft tissues: weakness in the intrinsic plantar muscles; overstretching of the long muscles of the sole of the foot; lengthening of the tendon of the tibialis posterior; overstretching of the ligaments and plantar fascia; shortening of the fibular muscles due to excessive pronation

Relationship to trunk rotation: trunk rotation to the left increases pronation of the right foot; trunk rotation to the right increases pronation of the left foot

TIP

In addition to lengthening of muscles, there is overstretching of ligaments and of the plantar fascia.

Lateral View

Other Observations

In this step, make any observations not yet recorded in the earlier steps for the lateral view of the lower half of the body, such as scars and bruising. For example, the person in figure 1.46 has edematous feet. Observe also the second toe of the right foot.

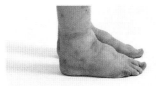

Figure 1.46 Example of edematous feet.
Courtesy of Emma Kelly Photography.

Quick Questions

1. When using the anterior view, which bony landmark is it useful to use when assessing someone for pelvic rotation?

2. Why is it more accurate to measure the Q angle with your client standing rather than supine?

3. When someone has a pelvis that is laterally tilted upwards on the right, which hip is adducted and which hip is abducted?

4. In the posterior view, what is the purpose of imagining or drawing a line down the midline of the calf?

5. What key observations might indicate to you that someone has genu recurvatum posture (knee hyperextension)?

Measuring the Effectiveness of Your Treatment

Learning Outcomes

After reading this chapter, you should be able to do the following:

- Recall examples of overall treatment aims.
- Develop specific treatment goals.
- Determine the most appropriate way to measure the effectiveness of your treatments.

Whenever you provide treatment to a client with a lower limb issue – whether this is the use of a hands-on technique, the prescription of exercises or the giving of advice, for example – you want to know whether it has been helpful. You need to ask yourself whether or not what you have provided to the client has been effective, because this will help to plan further treatment or to know when someone no longer needs treatment. With any form of therapy, it is vital to identify not only when something has worked but also when something has failed. It is important to acknowledge failure as well as success, because by doing this, you can identify barriers to recovery.

To determine whether something has been effective, you need to answer three questions:

1. What was the overall treatment aim?
2. What treatment was provided?
3. How are you going to measure effectiveness?

This chapter provides ideas for how to determine an overall treatment aim, set more specific treatment goals, and measure their outcomes.

Deciding on an Overall Treatment Aim

Before you can create a specific treatment goal, it is necessary to decide on an overall treatment aim. You may be thinking that the treatment aim is obvious: recovery from a hamstring strain, for example. However, it is helpful to break this down into more specific components, because by doing so, you create the foundation on which to base the goal of your treatment and measure its effectiveness. Examples of overall treatment aims are listed below.

Examples of Overall Treatment Aims

- Reduce pain
- Reduce swelling
- Improve balance
- Overcome the sensation of muscle stiffness
- Overcome or prevent muscle cramping
- Regain normal movement in a joint
- Improve weight bearing through the lower limb
- Improve lower limb strength
- Regain everyday lower limb function
- Educate the client
- Help correct postural imbalance

The overall aim is likely to be different for each client you are treating. For example, you could be treating someone recovering from a recent injury who has pain and swelling and is unable to walk, or you may be treating someone who has not been injured but suffers from persistent calf cramps. You may be treating someone who is managing a long-term condition such as osteoarthritis in the knee whose main aim is to maintain normal daily function, or perhaps you have been approached by someone waiting for surgery who has been advised to strengthen their legs in preparation. Use the list of suggested overall treatment aims to help you identify your main aim or treatment.

If you are treating someone over several weeks or months, it is important to return to this list periodically and ask whether the overall aim has changed, because this is likely to be the case. Your specific treatment goals will then need to be revised. Think of your treatment aim as a target, with the goals as specific steps you need to take to reach it.

Creating Specific Treatment Goals

Once you have identified the main aim of your treatment, the next step is to determine a more specific treatment goal. This is important because it helps you to measure the effectiveness of your treatment. Table 2.1 provides two examples for how each of the overall treatment aims listed previously might be developed into more specific goals. Please note that these are just a few examples and that there are many possible treatment goals relating to each general treatment aim.

Table 2.1   Developing Specific Lower Limb Treatment Goals

Examples of general treatment aims	Examples of specific treatment goals
Reduce pain	Over the next 2 weeks, reduce the severity and incidence of pain in the left knee from a daily 8 out of 10 on a numerical pain rating scale. Over the next 4 weeks, reduce the severity and incidence of pain in the right hip from 5 out of 10 on a visual analogue scale.
Reduce swelling	Over the next 24 hours, reduce swelling in the right ankle from an ankle girth circumference of 35.5 cm (14 in.). Over the next 2 days, reduce swelling in the left knee from a circumference of 43 cm (17 in.), measured at approximately the tibial tuberosity.
Improve balance	Over the next 3 weeks, be able to sway confidently from side to side from the left to right foot, maintaining contact with the floor. Within the next 10 days, progress from static right-leg standing to right-leg standing whilst brushing teeth, combing hair etc.
Overcome the sensation of muscle stiffness	Over the next 14 days, reduce the frequency and sensation of daily stiffness in the left hamstrings from 9 out of 10. Within the next 4 weeks, reduce the frequency and sensation of stiffness in both calves from a daily 5 out of 10.
Overcome or prevent muscle cramping	Over the next 7 days, reduce the frequency of cramping in the right calf and toes at night. Over the next 14 days, reduce the frequency of postexercise cramping in the left hamstrings.
Regain normal movement in a joint	Within the next 3 months, regain full extension in the left knee. Over the next 6 weeks, regain full active range of motion in the right ankle in all ranges.
Improve weight bearing through the lower limb	Over the next 2 weeks, be able to sit in a chair with both feet on the ground. Over the next 10 days, be able to bear weight fully through the right leg when standing.
Improve lower limb strength	Over the next 12 weeks, improve the strength of the left hip extensor muscles. Within the next 12 weeks, improve the strength of the right calf muscle.
Regain everyday lower limb function	Over the next 4 weeks, be able to walk 9 m (10 yd) without pain. Over the next 2 weeks, be able to alternate between sit-to-stand and stand-to-sit positions.
Educate the client	At the next treatment session, provide education regarding the condition of plantar fasciitis by using an anatomical model of a foot. At the next appointment, provide education regarding typical healing times after a lateral ankle sprain and the importance of a balance training programme.
Help correct postural imbalance	Perform a posterior pelvic tilt in the standing position using 1 set of 5 repetitions performed 3 times during the day. Daily, practise walking conscientiously for 3 minutes with a more neutral foot posture, avoiding the toe-in position.

Observe how each of the more specific goals begins with a time frame. Clients sometimes have a specific date in mind that marks the start of a holiday, a return to work, a birthday or an anniversary, so a specific date could be used, such as 'by the 28th of April'. Quite often, the time frame is determined according to the next appointment the person may have with you. For some people, having this kind of accountability can be helpful.

Usually, a treatment goal is developed in discussion with the client. Once they have agreed on a treatment goal, you can then determine how best this might be achieved. It is extremely important to create a recovery or maintenance programme that is customized to each client. For example, table 2.2 provides examples of three clients who have all sustained a confirmed moderate sprain to the lateral ligament of the ankle and contrasts their lifestyle and health behaviours. Assuming you had no other information than that provided in table 2.2, what are your immediate thoughts when you read these descriptions? Would you agree that these clients are likely to respond differently to treatment? What barriers do you perceive there to be? For example, is there anything that suggests the likelihood of compliance with an exercise programme?

Table 2.2   Contrasting Three Clients With a Moderate Lateral Ankle Sprain

Client	Health	Lifestyle and psychosocial factors
Aged 86: Sustained sprain when knocked into by someone on a skateboard in the park	Considers self to be in good health. Non-smoker. Reports osteoarthritis in both knees but says that this does not significantly impair function other than in the winter months, when pain is slightly increased and it takes longer to get dressed in the mornings. No previous ankle injuries.	For the past 5 years, has enjoyed participating in a daily yoga class that involves strength and mobility. Walks 40 minutes daily. Lives alone, independently. Describes being generally of a happy disposition. Reports growing up in 'war years' and states, 'It's just a sprain'. Is keen to recover in order to return to yoga. Wants to know which exercises are best for recovery. Has asked whether it would be OK to start tai chi classes.
Aged 51: Sustained sprain after slipping on liquid in the supermarket when shopping	Non-smoker. Hypertension. Prediabetic. Four ankle sprains to the same ankle over the past 4 years; says, 'It's my bad ankle'.	Sedentary worker. Never been physically active due to having a large family and lacking time. Has been thinking about losing weight. Was intending to start recreational cycling with family. Is considering starting swimming classes but is concerned about body size. Expects to sprain the ankle again, given the past history of this.
Aged 45: Tripped at work	Smoker. Hypertension. High cholesterol. Chronic low back pain. Pain in knees and both ankles, which doctor attributes to significant weight gain but which client disputes.	Manual worker. Believes work is to blame for the injury. Intends to seek compensation. Lives alone. Reports having been advised to exercise for the management of back and lower limb pain in the past but found this 'a waste of time' because 'I need a scan to know what's wrong'. Believes an orthotic boot should have been provided to wear after this ankle injury.

Determining the Most Appropriate Measure of Effectiveness

There are many different ways to measure the effectiveness of your treatment. Which measure you select depends on what your specific goal is. For example, if your goal is to reduce pain, then you would use a pain measurement scale, and if your goal is to improve a client's ability to perform an everyday function, then you would use a functional assessment scale. Examples of the different ways you could measure a treatment's effectiveness are described in this section. At the end of this chapter, you will find examples of pretreatment and posttreatment measurements used to determine the effectiveness of a treatment for trigger points in the gluteal muscles.

Measuring Pain

Pain is measured using self-report tools, the two most common being the Visual Analogue Scale (VAS) and the Numerical Pain Rating Scale (NPRS). Both of these scales have been adopted as recommended outcome measures by the Faculty of Pain Medicine and the British Pain Society (2019). The VAS is simply an unmarked horizontal line, with the left end signifying being pain free and the right end signifying the worst pain imaginable. The client marks the line according to how close to one end of the scale they rate their pain. The value of this scale is that it could be modified to record other sensations, such as stiffness, aching or discomfort. This scale can easily be quantified if the length of the line used matches a predetermined length. For example, if a line measuring 10 cm (4 in.) is drawn and the client marks the centre of the line, this equates to '5'; if they mark close to the right-hand side of the line, this might equate to '9'; if they mark close to the left-hand side, this might equate to '2'.

The NPRS is also a horizontal line, but it is different than the VAS in that it has the numbers 0 to 10 assigned to it at regular intervals: 0 on the left end of the line and 10 on the right end. The client marks the number that they believe represents their pain. For example, 6 would be recorded as 6 out of 10.

One thing to note about the use of pain scales is that they are often embedded within functional assessment scales. If you are using a functional assessment scale that includes a pain score, you would not need to also use the VAS or the NPRS.

Measuring Muscle Length

One of the best sources for information on testing the length of muscles is the book *Muscles: Testing and Function* (Kendall, McCreary, and Provance, 1993), which provides illustrations of how to test specific muscles. Common tests for the lower limb are the prone knee bend test (for the length of the quadriceps), the straight-leg raise test (for the length of the hamstrings), the Thomas test (for the length of the hip flexors) and the Ober test (for the length of the iliotibial band). A useful test for the length of the calf muscles is to have the client stand facing a wall and step one foot backwards, as if to do a calf stretch. Notice how far from the wall the heel reaches on that leg; repeat with the other leg and compare. The farther the heel is from the wall, the longer the calf muscles.

TIP

It is important to remember that it is impossible to isolate individual muscles because they are wrapped in fascia, and fascia is connected to other structures, including in the lower limb. Therefore, the measurement derived depends on multiple structures, and restrictions in length may be due to connecting structures as well as a muscle itself.

In very simple terms, on the posterior aspect of the body, the fascia of the sole of the foot, the calf and the hamstrings is connected, and this fascia in turn is connected to the gluteal muscles and lower back. On the anterior aspect, the fascia of the hip flexors is also connected to the abdomen above and to the shin below. This means that any technique used to lengthen a muscle is likely to have an effect on the soft tissues above and below it. For example, lengthening the tissues of the lower back and calf results in an improvement in the straight-leg raise test, even if no techniques are applied to the hamstrings.

Measuring Joint Range of Motion

For detailed information on using a goniometre and the ranges of motion considered typical in human joints, refer to *The Clinical Measurement of Joint Motion* (Greene and Heckman 1994). When assessing a joint, remember that many factors can limit the range of motion, including a restriction in the joint itself (such as the shape of the joint) and laxity or tightness in the soft tissues surrounding the joint. It is important to test the range of motion both passively and actively. A passive test might reveal that a person has a good range of motion that would otherwise be difficult to determine when assessed actively, because active movements could be limited by pain or lack of strength.

Measuring Function

There are many different functional assessment scales, and some of these have been developed specifically for the assessment of lower limb conditions. For example, Binkley and colleagues (1999) developed the Lower Extremity Functional Scale. This simple scale asks users to score the level of difficulty they have, or would have, if attempting certain activities, irrespective of what lower limb condition they have. The kinds of activities listed include putting on shoes, sitting for an hour, walking between rooms and getting out of a bath. In a systematic review, Mehta and colleagues (2016) found this scale to be valid and reliable for assessing a wide range of patients with lower extremity musculoskeletal conditions. Other functional assessment scales have been developed specific to the hamstrings, knee, ankle and foot. Some of these are described in the following section.

Functional Assessment Tools

Hamstrings

The Hamstring Outcome Score is a 5-domain questionnaire that assesses an athlete's soreness, symptoms, pain, activities (sports) and quality of life. Questions are scored from 0 to 4, from no complaints to maximum complaints. A score of 100% suggests no complaints in all domains. A score of 80% or more indicates a low risk for hamstring strain injury, whereas a score below 80% indicates a high risk for hamstring strain injury. This tool can also be used as a predictor of future hamstring injuries (van de Hoef et al. 2021).

Another useful scale is the Functional Assessment Scale for Acute Hamstring Injuries. This is a reliable and validated 10-item questionnaire used to assess function after an acute hamstring injury (Malliaropoulos et al. 2014). Additionally, clinical practice guidelines that summarise the best evidence for the assessment of and outcome measures for hamstring strain are provided by Martin and colleagues (2022).

Knee

A useful tool for measuring knee function is the Knee Injury and Osteoarthritis Outcome Score. This tool encompasses 5 different subscales: pain, symptoms, activities of daily living, sport and recreational function and quality of life. The composite of these scores is measured on a scale of 100, with 0 being extreme knee dysfunction and 100 being no knee dysfunction. Roos and Lohmander (2003) provide a helpful review of this measurement tool.

A useful tool for assessing people with knee problems is the International Knee Documentation Committee Subjective Knee Form (Irrgang et al. 2001). This can be used to evaluate people with problems of the meniscus or knee ligaments, patellofemoral dysfunction and osteoarthritis. The form is used to assess a person's subjective responses to questions such as the highest level of activity they can perform without significant knee pain and other questions related to swelling and locking of the knee.

The Knee Society Knee Scoring System is another assessment tool that is specifically designed for use before and after knee replacement surgery. This measurement tool includes both subjective and objective (knee alignment, instability and joint motion) measurements. It includes a patient's perception of everyday activities such as standing, walking and using stairs as well as a range of physical recreational and sporting activities that may be important to them. Scuderi and colleagues (2012) provide a detailed description of this system.

Foot and Ankle

If you were treating someone with plantar fasciitis, it would be appropriate to use a questionnaire such as the Plantar Fasciitis Pain and Disability Scale questionnaire. Willis and colleagues (2009) found this to be a useful way to differentiate between pain due to plantar fasciitis and heel pain from other causes.

The Ankle Osteoarthritis Scale (Domsic and Saltzman 1998) uses a simple scoring method to measure pain when performing everyday activities and the perceived difficulty in performing everyday activities in people with osteoarthritis in the ankle. Many of the functional assessment tools for the ankle involve hopping and jumping, because these test strength, balance and coordination. For example, Madsen, Hall and Docherty (2018) provided a useful example of a test for assessing outcomes in people with chronic ankle instability. Their study used a simple hopping test and measured the time it took to perform the test, the distance hopped and the participant's perceived

(continued)

Functional Assessment Tools *(continued)*

amount of ankle instability. You may, however, be treating someone who is unable to hop, and there is nothing wrong with assessing less strenuous everyday activities such as walking, climbing stairs or standing from a sitting position. You might even decide that simply asking a person to rate their perceived effort in transferring weight from one limb to the other is sufficient in the early stages of rehabilitation.

Examples of Pretreatment and Posttreatment Measurements

Huguenin and colleagues (2005) examined the effect of dry needling trigger points in the gluteal muscles during the straight-leg raise test and internal rotation of the hip. They randomly assigned 59 male runners to a group that received dry needling to trigger points in the gluteal muscles or a group that received placebo needling to trigger points. Triggers were reported in most participants to be in the upper outer buttock quadrant and were pierced by the dry needle in one group, but in the placebo group, the needle only touched the skin without piercing it. The straight-leg raise test and internal rotation of the hip were measured at baseline, immediately after the intervention and at 24 and 72 hours after the intervention by taking digital photographs of the test positions. Visual analogue scale scores were also recorded. There was no significant change in VAS scores or gluteal pain after running, but both groups showed significant improvement in reported hamstring tightness, hamstring pain and gluteal tightness after running. The authors commented that the results could indicate one of three things: (1) The postulated restriction in range of motion measured by the straight-leg raise test and internal rotation test may not be associated with symptoms, (2) dry needling had no effect on muscle length in these muscles or (3) the outcome measures used were not appropriate to measure change resulting from dry needling of trigger points.

Quick Questions

1. What is the difference between a treatment aim and a treatment goal?
2. List five of the treatment aims mentioned in this chapter.
3. Name the two pain measurement tools described in this chapter.
4. Using the information in this chapter, list four common tests used to assess the length of lower limb muscles.
5. What is the Lower Extremity Functional Scale, and how is it scored?

PART II

Hands-On Techniques for Common Muscular Problems

This part of the book concentrates on hands-on techniques, such as massage, trigger point release, soft tissue release (STR) and taping, which can be used to help address common musculoskeletal conditions affecting the lower limb. Passive and active stretches are included too.

There are four chapters within this part of the book. Chapter 3 covers conditions affecting the gluteal, groin and hip flexor muscles. Chapter 4 describes conditions affecting the thigh – specifically, the hamstrings and quadriceps. In chapter 5, you will learn how to use hands-on techniques to help clients with knee, calf and shin problems, and for clients with problems in their ankles and feet, you will find information in chapter 6. With almost all conditions, it is important to maintain or regain strength and balance in the affected body part and in the lower limb in general, and part III is devoted to this specialised topic. Within chapters 3 through 6, you will be directed to the chapters with relevant material related to strengthening.

In a few cases, the order of the techniques provided is arbitrary. In many cases, however, the techniques most likely to be most effective are described first. For example, in a case of acute injury, active techniques are preferable to passive ones simply because there is reduced likelihood of reinjury, and when treating chronic conditions, passive techniques are valuable in jump-starting the rehabilitation process. However, in all cases, it is important to reduce the client's reliance on you and increase their active participation in recovery. If a client has become used to long-term hands-on treatment, this can be a challenge.

As with other titles in the Hands-On Guides for Therapists series, in *Soft Tissue Therapy for the Lower Limb,* material has been organised by compartmentalising the body. This is for ease of description. You are most likely reading this book as someone who has hands-on therapy skills or whose training involves these skills. You will therefore know that when treating someone, we need to view them holistically and that a condition in one part of the body almost always affects another part of the body.

Gluteal, Groin and Hip Flexor Muscles

Learning Outcomes

After reading this chapter, you should be able to do the following:

- Apply trigger point release to the gluteal muscles and hip flexors.
- Use the forearms, fists or elbows as appropriate when applying massage to treat piriformis syndrome, groin strain and tight hip adductors.
- Apply soft tissue release strategies to the gluteal muscles and hip flexors.
- Use passive stretches to stretch the gluteal muscles, hip adductors and hip flexors.
- Explain which active stretches might be most appropriate for the gluteal muscles, hip adductors and hip flexors.

In this chapter, you will learn how to help clients with trigger points in the gluteal muscles, piriformis syndrome, groin strain, tight hip adductors and tight hip flexors using massage, trigger point release, soft tissue release (STR) and both active and passive stretching. In almost all cases, strengthening is valuable for assisting recovery, whether this is to regain strength in the muscle itself or to strengthen an opposing muscle group for reciprocal inhibition. People with an acute injury often compensate by overusing the opposite limb; people with a condition affecting their right hip, for example, commonly have pain in their left knee. Reducing the pain of a hip condition is therefore important because it can help a person to regain a proper gait pattern before compensation has a detrimental effect on the hip and knee joints. Chapter 7 contains examples of helpful exercises to strengthen the hip. Because hip conditions also affect the rest of the lower limb, you may discover that your client has issues in their knee or even their ankle, and chapters 4, 5 and 6 may also be helpful.

Trigger Points in the Gluteal Muscles

Trigger Point Release

Trigger points are found throughout all three gluteal muscles – in the gluteus maximus close to the lateral border of the sacrum, in the gluteus medius running inferior to the iliac crest and in the gluteus minimus. Trigger points in the gluteal muscles are aggravated by prolonged immobility, either when sitting or standing, and they are associated with trigger points in the quadratus lumborum muscle. Some of the gluteal trigger points are illustrated in figure 3.1 with white circles.

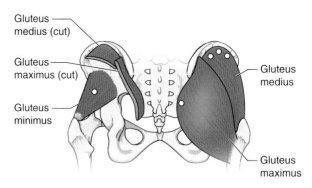

Figure 3.1   Trigger points in the gluteal muscles.

The gluteus maximus trigger point causes pain along the sacroiliac joint and into the base of the buttock on that side, and it is easy to identify when your client is in a side-lying position. The gluteus maximus is also associated with trigger points in the hamstrings and lumbar erector spinae; pain is perpetuated by prolonged sitting and activities that require hip and spine extension, such as repeated lifting of a heavy object.

The trigger points in the gluteus medius cause pain in the sacrum, sacroiliac joint and ipsilateral (same-side) buttock. Palpate for these triggers when your client is in either the side-lying or the prone position, sliding your fingers inferiorly off the iliac crest. Trigger points in the gluteus medius, perhaps more than in the other two gluteal muscles, are perpetuated by gait abnormalities, as might be caused by leg-length discrepancy or Morton foot (in which the second toe is longer than the big toe). They are also aggravated by prolonged sitting and prolonged hip flexion.

Trigger points are found throughout the upper portion of the gluteus minimus and cause pain in the buttock and lateral thigh and leg on that side. To palpate these trigger points, position your client supine, locate the tensor fasciae latae, and work your fingers posteriorly into the gluteus minimus. Because it is a deep muscle, you are unlikely to be able to identify specific triggers easily, but you may be able to reproduce mild tenderness when applying pressure here.

Onik and colleagues (2020) conducted an interesting study of myofascial trigger points in the gluteal region that they had identified using both palpation and thermal imaging. Their study involved 30 participants who were asked to rank pretreatment and posttreatment trigger point pain that was reproducible on palpation, using a numerical rating scale. Treatment consisted of simple progressive compression of a trigger point for

1 minute. All participants reported a significant reduction in posttreatment pain and had an initial increase in skin surface temperature, followed by a decrease. The researchers postulated that after compression of the trigger point, there was local occlusion of blood to the area, followed by vasodilation once the pressure was released. They were reluctant to speculate as to the reasons for this; however, their study provides a useful contribution to the understanding of trigger points.

TIP

Using Gentle Pressure to Release Trigger Points

A great way to alleviate tension in the gluteal area is simply to compress the tissues, focusing on areas of tightness. You can do this using your forearm or elbow. Start by working over the area consistently with your forearm, avoiding the use of your elbows. Figure 3.2 illustrates the procedure (the client shown in the figure is more side-lying than three-quarter lying; however, three-quarter lying will give you better access to the gluteal muscles). You can continue to treat the area in this way, or you can apply a little oil, place a towel over the area, and work through the towel. The oil will grip the towel, and you can use a twisting movement to stretch and compress the tissues. This is a nice alternative to treating the gluteal muscles in the prone position and can be combined with treatment to the lateral thigh of the limb and the tensor fasciae latae muscle on the same side.

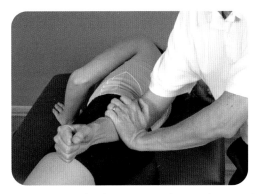

Figure 3.2   Gentle pressure using the forearm to release trigger points.

TIP

A mistake some therapists make when treating gluteal muscles is to use too much pressure too soon in too precise an area. In the three-quarter lying position, the client will sense the pressure far more than when prone.

With the client positioned as for figure 3.2, use your elbows as a way to focus pressure to more defined areas. Start by leaning onto the client, using your forearm to gauge their sensitivity to pressure. Should the client require deeper pressure, slowly flex your elbow (figure 3.3). Remember that you need to flex your elbow only a few degrees for the client to experience a disproportionate rise in pressure. This technique is a great way to focus pressure to localised areas. However, this area is highly sensitive to pressure in many people, so apply this technique cautiously.

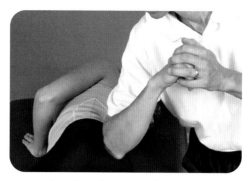

Figure 3.3 Gentle pressure using the elbow to release trigger points.

TIP

In whichever treatment position you are using (prone, side-lying or three-quarter lying), be aware of deep pressure to the piriformis muscle, because this can be painful. Note that discomfort does not necessarily indicate piriformis syndrome, as is believed by some therapists.

You can teach clients how to release trigger points themselves. To do this, have them stand with their back to a wall and place a ball between the buttock on one side and the wall (figure 3.4).

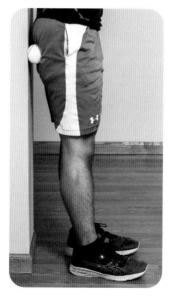

Figure 3.4 Positioning a ball to self-release trigger points in the gluteal muscles.

Stretching

Figure 3.5 (*a, b*) provides examples of active stretches that are useful after trigger point release. The passive stretch shown in figure 3.5*c* is useful but difficult to apply with a client on a treatment couch because of the force needed to stretch the strong muscles of the buttock region. To perform the passive stretch, start with the client's hip and knee at a 90-degree angle, as shown, and move the lower limb towards the client in an attempt to stretch the gluteal region. Solicit feedback from the client to help determine the best position to hold the stretch. Some clients find this position uncomfortable when it compresses the rectus femoris tendon on the anterior of the hip.

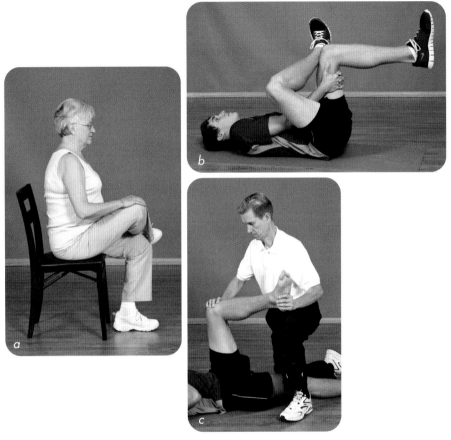

Figure 3.5 *(a, b)* Active and *(c)* passive stretches for gluteal muscles after deactivation of trigger points.

Soft Tissue Release

Soft tissue release can be used successfully to release trigger points in the gluteal muscles too. It can be done with your client in the side-lying position or prone. Two methods are described here.

With experimentation, it is possible to locate the fibres of the gluteus minimus with your client in the side-lying position. Trigger points in this muscle can be more difficult to access when using STR in the prone position. You may find that you need to lower your treatment couch to make working with the side-lying client easier, because their body will be higher than when they rest prone or supine. When you begin, it is challenging to keep a client balanced in the side-lying position whilst you focus your lock in the correct spot on the muscles. With practice, you will be able to identify triggers in the gluteus maximus and use STR in this position to deactivate them. With your client in the side-lying position and the hip in neutral, use your forearm (close to the elbow) to lock the gluteal muscles, directing your pressure towards the sacrum (figure 3.6a). Whilst maintaining your lock, ask your client to flex the hip, perhaps by asking them to take the knee to the chest (figure 3.6b). Repeat this action for a few minutes, varying the position of your lock and working on the area that feels most beneficial for the client.

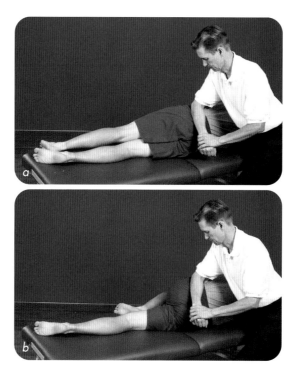

Figure 3.6 *(a)* Locking the gluteal muscles close to the sacrum with the hip in a neutral position followed by *(b)* active hip flexion.

TIP

It is quite challenging to apply active assisted STR to the gluteal muscles, and it takes practice to focus your lock in the correct spot on the muscles. With experience, however, you will discover a small area that, when locked, provides for the greatest degree of stretch.

Another way to apply STR to the gluteal muscles is with your client in the prone position. Grasp the ankle of the leg closest to you and flex the knee. Gently lock the tissues using your elbow, fist or thumb. In figure 3.7a, the therapist has chosen to use the elbow to lock fibres of the gluteus medius. Maintaining your lock, rotate the femur by passively moving the ankle towards you or away from you, experimenting to determine where your client feels the stretch most (figure 3.7b).

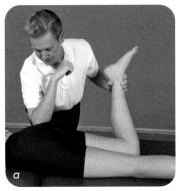
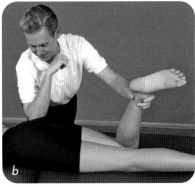

Figure 3.7 *(a)* Gently locking the gluteal muscles with an elbow, then *(b)* passively rotating the femur whilst locking the tissues of the buttock to bring about a stretch.

One way for your client to perform STR on the gluteal muscles is to use a tennis ball (figure 3.8a), just as they did for simple trigger point release, but then to flex their hip (figure 3.8b). Because this technique requires standing on one leg as the hip is flexed, it can be difficult for people with poor balance.

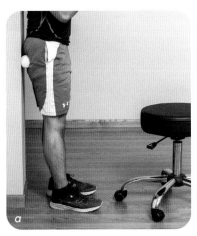
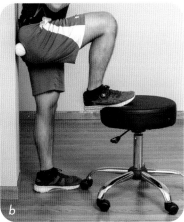

Figure 3.8 *(a)* Static pressure to the gluteal muscles using a tennis ball followed by *(b)* active hip flexion brings about a stretch in the gluteal muscles.

TIP

To stretch the gluteus medius and minimus, the client could change their position so that their back is turned away from the wall or they are standing almost with the side of their body to the wall as they not only flex but adduct the hip. Try this for yourself. Notice how medial rotation of the hip can bring about a stretch in some parts of the gluteal muscles once you have locked them using a ball.

Piriformis Syndrome

Piriformis syndrome is the name given to pain in the buttocks and lower limb resulting from compression of the sciatic nerve in the region of the piriformis muscle, perhaps caused by the muscle itself. As the sciatic nerve runs from the sacrum and down the lower limb, it passes above, below or through the piriformis muscle. When piriformis syndrome results from compression of the nerve by the piriformis muscle, you have the opportunity to reduce symptoms. Some therapists erroneously believe that if they position the client into a side-lying pose and press the midregion of the buttock, the resulting pain indicates piriformis syndrome or trigger points. It is certainly possible to access the region of the piriformis muscle with the client in the side-lying position, but unsurprisingly, localised pressure here will be painful, as this is precisely how to access the sciatic nerve.

Clients with piriformis syndrome are likely to have a positive hip flexion, adduction and internal rotation sign, and this test can be helpful in determining treatment. Importantly, pain in this region can result from other conditions, such as spinal stenosis, and people with a poor response to treatment should be referred to a doctor.

Massage

It can be helpful to address trigger points in the surrounding muscles instead of attempting to massage the piriformis itself. As mentioned, the sciatic nerve is sensitive in many clients because of its proximity to the piriformis muscle, and if your pressure is too deep when massaging, clients will simply contract their muscles, defeating your efforts. The trick with massage to the region is to work the area within the client's pain threshold without causing spasm in the muscles.

Trigger Point Release

Trigger point release to the gluteal muscles using the techniques previously described is helpful at reducing tension in surrounding soft tissues.

Soft Tissue Release

Soft tissue release to the gluteal muscles as previously described is useful in reducing tension in the gluteal region.

Stretching

Both passive and active stretches are helpful to reduce pain from compression of the sciatic nerve in the piriformis region. The rationale for the use of stretching is twofold: to increase the resting length of the piriformis muscle and to reduce pressure on the sciatic nerve. The stretches shown in figure 3.5 are all appropriate. Unfortunately, whether performed actively or passively, the stretch initially tenses the muscle, and this in turn can compress the nerve, appearing to aggravate symptoms. Therefore, it is necessary to gradually build up the client's tolerance to stretching; otherwise, you risk turning them off to the use of this treatment.

Gulledge and colleagues (2014) conducted a study of the effectiveness of piriformis stretching among seven women diagnosed with piriformis syndrome. Three computed tomography scans were taken of participants who stretched their piriformis muscle before the second and third scans using stretches lasting 20 to 30 seconds repeated over a 5-minute period, for a total of 7 to 14 stretches. Gentle overpressure was used to a point at which the stretch was still tolerable. Gulledge and colleagues identified a 15% increase in the length of the piriformis after stretching. They reported that the most effective position for stretching this muscle was by placing the hip joint either in 115 degrees of hip flexion, 40 degrees of external rotation and 25 degrees of adduction or in 120 degrees of hip flexion, 50 degrees of external rotation and 30 degrees of adduction.

Strengthening

In piriformis syndrome, there is often atrophy of the gluteal muscles. It is therefore very important to engage your client in a programme of gluteal strengthening. Please see chapter 7 for more information.

Sitting Habits

Prolonged sitting is likely to be an aggravating factor in people with piriformis syndrome. Therefore, it will be important to work with your client to introduce short, frequent breaks if sitting is part of their occupation or to change their behaviour if prolonged sitting is habitual.

Groin Strain

Groin strains are particularly common in sports where muscles such as the adductor longus or the gracilis may be damaged by impact, sudden contraction or overstretching. There is pain on palpation of the insertion of the adductors at the pubis and pain on both resisted adduction and on stretching these muscles.

Acute Stage

All forms of deep massage and stretching should be avoided during the early stages of tissue repair.

Sub-Acute Stage

In the sub-acute stage, massage to the adductors could be applied with the client in the supine position. With a low treatment couch, position your client so that the thigh is gently abducted and supported on your thigh, as shown in figure 3.9a. Use a folded towel under the client's leg (figure 3.9b) for support, if necessary. To treat the left adductors, use your left arm. Starting just above the knee, glide your forearm slowly across the adductors towards the groin.

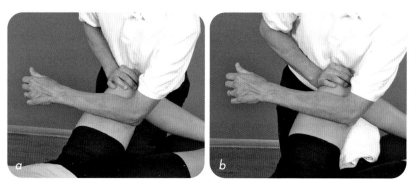

Figure 3.9 (a) Using your forearm to gently massage the adductors; (b) using a towel for support.

Massage

Working with your client in the three-quarter lying position, you can access the adductors of the limb when it is against the plinth. For example, to treat the right adductor muscles, have your client lie on their right side, with the adductors clearly exposed. One way to achieve this is for the client to flex their left hip, bringing the knee of that hip to rest on the plinth. Taking care not to press into the popliteal space at the back of the knee, gently rest your forearm on the client and slowly but firmly glide towards the ischium (figure 3.10). Take care to protect your posture when leaning forwards to apply pressure.

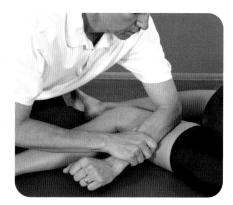

Figure 3.10 Massage the adductors using the forearm.

Stretching

Stretching should be conservative to prevent reinjuring muscles not yet fully healed. Groin strains can take a long time to heal; therefore, implementation of an early active stretching programme is recommended, providing this does not cause pain. Passive stretches are not recommended for groin strains, but many varieties of active stretches may be used.

Lying on a bed or the floor, a client could begin by gently abducting the legs (with the knees extended). If this is tolerable, they could progress to sitting cross-legged (figure 3.11a), placing pillows beneath each knee for support if there is discomfort. Once this position is tolerable, they could progress to the position in figure 3.11b, with the soles of the feet touching. To increase the stretch in either position, the client can simply place gentle downward pressure on the knees.

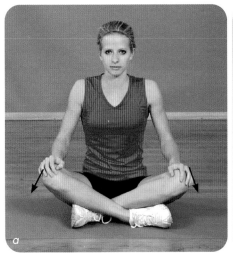 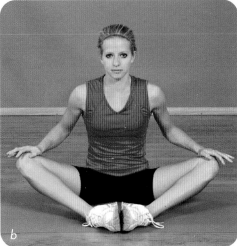

Figure 3.11 Progressing an active groin stretch from *(a)* the cross-legged position to *(b)* the sole-touching position, perhaps with overpressure on the knees.

An alternative adductor stretch is shown in figure 3.12. To increase this stretch, the client simply leans forwards; to decrease it, they lean backwards. Note that this stretch also requires flexibility in the hamstrings.

Strengthening

Strengthening of the adductor muscles is extremely important for preventing further groin strains. Chapter 7 provides detailed information about this.

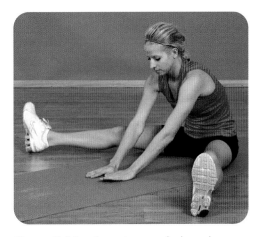

Figure 3.12 A groin stretch that also requires hamstring flexibility.

Tight Hip Adductors

People who engage in sporting activities such as running, football and swimming often find it is beneficial to stretch their adductor muscles as part of their cooldown programme of stretches or simply to decrease sensations of stiffness after exercise. Adductors contract as we walk, so people who walk a lot as part of their general lifestyle or fitness activities may also benefit from stretching these muscles. Adductors may become tight after periods of immobility, leading to muscle imbalance in the pelvis and lower limbs.

Massage

Warming the tissues using the forearm in either the supine (figure 3.13a) or side-lying (figure 3.13b) position is appropriate. To apply deeper pressure, you could use your fists (figure 3.13c), and for more specific work, you could use your elbow (figure 3.13d) to target specific tissues.

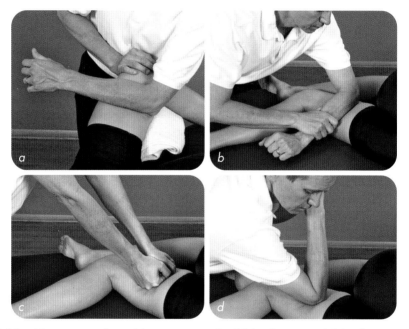

Figure 3.13 Massage to the adductors using (a, b) the forearm, (c) the fists, or (d) an elbow.

Stretching

Useful passive adductor stretches are shown in figure 3.14. Notice how in figure 3.14a, the therapist prevents the pelvis from moving by gently placing pressure on the anterior superior iliac spine. This can be uncomfortable for some clients, so you might want to place a sponge or small towel between your hand and the client's hip. In figure 3.14b, the therapist is abducting the leg whilst being sure to support the knee. Notice that in this position, extension of the lumbar spine may be exaggerated, and this is a position that may aggravate back pain in some clients.

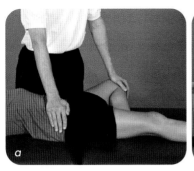 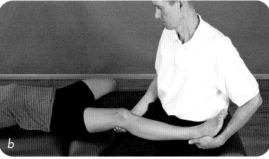

Figure 3.14 (a) Passive stretch to adductors of the left hip by stabilising the pelvis and applying gentle pressure to the right anterior superior iliac spine and (b) passive stretch to adductors of the right hip with the knee supported in extension.

TIP

Notice how in figure 3.14b, the leg that is not being stretched has been hooked over one side of the treatment couch. This prevents the client from being pulled to one side of the couch. First check that this position is comfortable, and perhaps insert a sponge between the client's knee and the side of the couch.

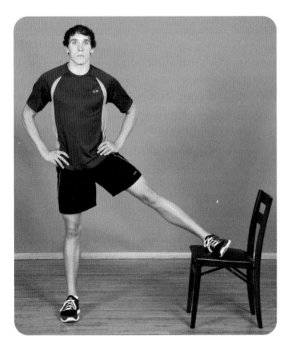

Each of the stretches in the groin strain section are helpful for combatting tight adductors. Other stretches include those shown in figures 3.15 and 3.16. Obviously, the stretch shown in figure 3.15 is not suitable for clients with balance problems, and the stretch shown in figure 3.16 places pressure on the knee of the leg not being stretched, so it is not suitable for all clients. Both of these stretches are safe, but bear in mind that they place more pressure on the medial collateral ligaments of the knee than the stretches shown in figure 3.11.

Figure 3.15 A standing adductor stretch.

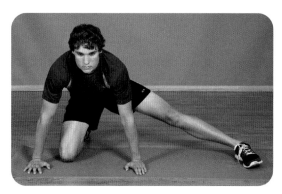

Figure 3.16 A kneeling adductor stretch.

Strengthening

Strengthening of the opposing muscle group – in this case, the hip abductor muscles – is beneficial. Chapter 7 describes specific gluteal strengthening exercises that may be helpful.

Tight Hip Flexors

The hip flexors include the psoas, iliacus, rectus femoris and tensor fasciae latae, all of which may feel tight after prolonged hip flexion or sporting activity. Because the rectus femoris is one of the quadriceps muscles, you would also benefit from reading about how to treat tight quadriceps in chapter 4.

A common belief among therapists is that people with shortened hip flexors will have reduced strength in the gluteal muscles, which could impair sporting performance, for example. However, Calvillo, Escalante and Kolber (2021) did not find this to be the case. Using techniques such as stretching to increase length in the hip flexors may therefore have little impact on gluteal strength, should that be your goal. Nonetheless, the material in this section will be useful for other reasons, such as for treating clients who report discomfort due to tension in their hip flexors or in whom you believe that hip flexor tension may be contributing to anterior pelvic tilt and potentially to low back pain. Reducing tension in the hip flexors may also be helpful in preventing injury: Tight hip flexors have been identified as a significant risk factor for hamstring injury in older adults who play Australian football (Gabbe, Bennell, and Finch 2006).

Trigger Point Release

A trigger point in the iliacus is located high in the muscle, just inferior to the iliac crest on the anterior of the ilium (figure 3.17). It sends pain down the upper part of the anterior thigh. Palpate for it with your client in the side-lying position, hooking your fingers gently over the crest and pressing them towards you (figure 3.18a). Prolonged hip flexion aggravates this trigger, which is associated with triggers in the psoas and quadratus lumborum muscles. Ferguson (2014) provides three case studies of clients with idiopathic scoliosis, describing how trigger points in muscles, including the iliacus, affect and are affected by spine shape.

Oh and colleagues (2016) describe how an inflatable ball was used to deactivate triggers in a range of muscles, including the iliacus, in a group of older patients with chronic low back pain. All participants had trigger points in the gluteus maximus, gluteus medius, iliopsoas and quadratus lumborum on at least

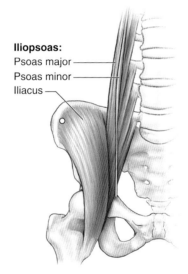

Iliopsoas:
Psoas major
Psoas minor
Iliacus

Figure 3.17 Trigger point in the iliacus.

one side that had persisted for more than 2 months. The iliopsoas was treated actively with the patients in the prone position; the hip on the affected side was abducted to approximately 45 degrees, and the knee was flexed to 90 degrees. Significant improvements were found in pain scores on the Visual Analogue Scale, pressure pain sensitivity and lumbar flexion.

Some clients may find this technique invasive; therefore, show your client where you intend to place your hands, and be sure to obtain the client's approval before performing this stretch. With your client in the side-lying position with the hip flexed, lock into the iliacus on the anterior surface of the ilium (figure 3.18a). The abdomen falls away in the side-lying position, so having the client in this position rather than supine is relatively safer. Whilst maintaining your lock, ask your client to straighten the leg, which extends the hip (figure 3.18b). The area to be worked is small, so the lock may be repeated in the same place or a centimetre to one side. Usually, performing the stretch three times this way will provide some relief from tension in the hip area.

If the client requires a greater degree of stretch, have them extend their hip at the end of the movement rather than pressing more firmly with your fingers. One way to explain this action is to ask the client to press into your fingers when you get to the end of the movement.

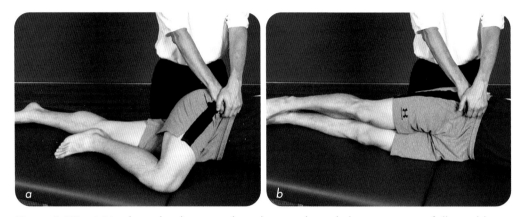

Figure 3.18 (a) Locking the iliacus with a client in the side-lying position, followed by (b) active hip extension as the lock is maintained by the therapist.

TIP

This area can be ticklish. An alternative approach is to ask the client to place their own hand on the area, and then you press over it. You can also dissipate your pressure by working through a facecloth folded into fourths.

It is always useful to explore whether there are trigger points in the tensor fasciae latae (figure 3.19). Locate this muscle by asking your client to raise their leg off the treatment couch, rotating it internally. Once you find the muscle, position a massage tool gently against it (figure 3.20). Press firmly into the muscle, searching for trigger spots. When you locate one, apply gentle pressure for 60 seconds, allowing the 'grateful pain' to dissipate. This is a great technique to save therapists' thumbs when deep pressure needs to be applied to this small muscle. Using a massage tool safely and effectively takes some practice; take care to avoid pressure to the greater trochanter.

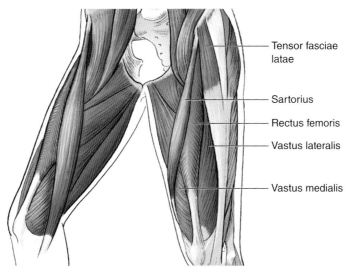

Tensor fasciae latae

Sartorius

Rectus femoris

Vastus lateralis

Vastus medialis

Figure 3.19   The tensor fasciae latae and its relationship to the quadriceps.

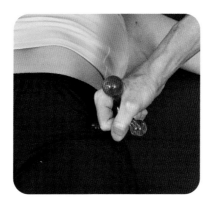

Figure 3.20   Treating trigger points in the tensor fasciae latae using a massage tool.

TIP

To identify the tensor fasciae latae, position the client supine and palpate the iliac crest. The muscle originates from the posterior aspect of the crest and will contract if you have the client lift their leg off the treatment couch and rotate the hip internally. (You can try this yourself whilst standing: Flex your hip and internally rotate it, keeping your knee straight.)

Stretching

Passive stretches for the hip flexors could be performed in the prone (figure 3.21) or supine (figure 3.22) position. To perform the stretch with the client prone, insert a small towel beneath the knee to take the hip into slight extension. In some clients, this increases lordosis in the lumbar spine and may be uncomfortable. Stretching the rectus femoris muscle in the prone position could be harmful if a client has a history of trauma to the low back, because the lumbar spine extends in this position. One way to reduce lumbar extension is for clients to perform a posterior pelvic tilt whilst you retain the position of the leg; thus, they perform the stretch themselves without your needing to flex the knee farther. This is also a good starting position for using Muscle Energy Technique (MET). An alternative is to place your hand on the pelvis before flexing the knee, preventing movement in the pelvis and spine.

Notice that in figure 3.22, the client needs to be positioned so that they are able to extend the hip (thereby stretching the hip flexors) and not have the thigh supported, as shown in the photograph.

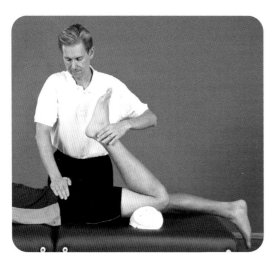

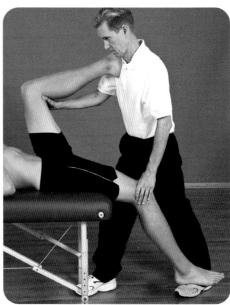

Figure 3.21   Using a towel increases extension of the hip and therefore facilitates hip flexor stretching in the prone position.

Figure 3.22   Hip flexor stretching in the supine position.

It is important to have a variety of stretches you can demonstrate for clients who have tight hip flexors. For example, figure 3.23 illustrates how to stretch the hip flexors by hanging the affected leg off one side of a bed. Kneeling (figure 3.24) is an alternative for clients who are comfortable on their knees. In both positions, flattening the low back so the pelvis is posteriorly tilted increases the stretch on the hip flexors. An easy way to explain this is to suggest that the client contract the buttock muscles. The stretch shown in figure 3.24 can be further enhanced if the client raises their arm above their head and turns towards the flexed knee of the opposite leg (figure 3.25). In this way, all the fasciae connecting the anterior hip and thigh and the lateral side of the body are tensioned.

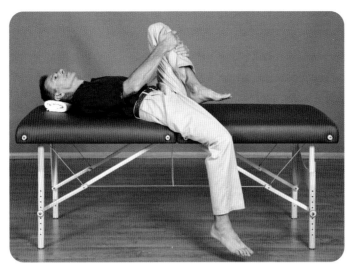

Figure 3.23   A supine hip flexor stretch.

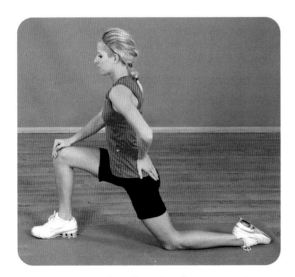

Figure 3.24   A kneeling hip flexor stretch.

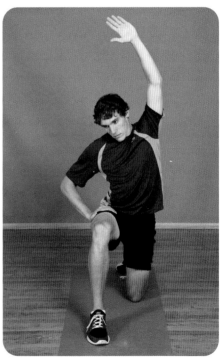

Figure 3.25   Enhancing a kneeling hip flexor stretch.

Strengthening

Due to reciprocal inhibition, strengthening of the opposing muscle group – in this case, the hip extensor muscles – is likely to be beneficial in reducing tension in the hip flexors. Chapter 7 has more information.

Quick Questions

1. Which nerve is affected in piriformis syndrome?

2. What are three ways the adductor muscles may be damaged in a groin strain?

3. If you wanted to apply a gentle passive stretch in the supine position to someone with tight left hip adductors, where would you position your right hand to stabilise the pelvis?

4. When treating someone with tight hip flexors, you decide to apply soft tissue release to the iliacus. In which treatment position do you apply this technique: prone, supine or side-lying?

5. How do you identify the tensor fasciae latae with a client in the supine position?

Hamstrings
and Quadriceps

4

Learning Outcomes

After reading this chapter, you should be able to do the following:

- Explain why active rather than passive techniques are the most appropriate intervention in the treatment of an acute hamstring strain.
- Demonstrate passive stretches for the hamstrings and quadriceps.
- Use the forearms, fists or elbows, as appropriate, when applying trigger point release to the hamstrings and quadriceps.
- Teach active stretches for the hamstrings and quadriceps.
- Apply soft tissue release to the hamstrings and quadriceps.

This chapter focuses on four common conditions affecting the hamstring and quadriceps muscles. You will learn which hands-on techniques might be most appropriate for hamstring strains and cramps and how to best help clients who report tension in these muscles. You will also learn how to deactivate trigger points in the hamstrings and quadriceps and which active and passive stretches are helpful. Strengthening exercises are important after a hamstring strain; chapter 7 explains how to do these.

Hamstring Strain

Tears to hamstring muscles are common and frequently involve the proximal musculotendinous junction of the biceps femoris. Strains are classified as mild, moderate or severe. In mild strains, few muscle fibres are torn. Moderate strains cause damage to more fibres and a distinct loss of function. When the strain is severe, complete rupture of the muscle occurs. In addition to being very painful, moderate to severe strains are extremely disabling. In all cases, there is pain on palpation, pain on stretching of the muscle and pain on resisted knee flexion or resisted hip extension. In severe cases, there is bruising and loss of strength in knee flexion or hip extension. A systematic review by Green and colleagues (2020) provides useful information about risk factors for hamstring strain injury. However, there is inconclusive evidence regarding the most effective interventions for a hamstring strain. A systematic review by Prior, Guerin and Grimmer (2009) provides a clear discussion of this topic.

Acute Stage

Deep tissue massage and all forms of stretching are avoided during the early stages of tissue repair after a hamstring strain, when protection of the damaged tissues is the goal of treatment.

Sub-Acute Stage

With a strain to any muscle, it is important to remember that pain subsides long before the healing process is complete. It is therefore wise to treat the client conservatively during the sub-acute phase of a hamstring strain, when there may be decreased pain and swelling. During this phase of recovery, the treatment aims are to minimise loss of hamstring strength and loss of range of motion in the hip and knee joints.

Massage

In the sub-acute stage of a hamstring strain, light effleurage superior to the site of the tear could be helpful in aiding lymphatic drainage, but deep tissue massage should be avoided. Begin with exploratory massage, using your fingertips to identify areas of adhesion. Using your forearms (figure 4.1) is an easy way to deliver broad strokes, which, along with stretching, can help collagen fibres realign in a more optimal way than they otherwise might. Whilst supporting yourself in flexion at the waist, position your forearm just above the knee. Use your left forearm if treating the client's right hamstrings. Lean onto the client and glide gently up to the ischium. End your stroke at the point on the thigh that is appropriate for your client. In sport massage, it is common to take the stroke all the way to the origin of the hamstrings at the ischium. For you to fully access these muscles, either your client will need to wear short shorts or you will need to provide towel draping.

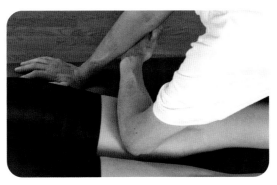

Figure 4.1   Gentle effleurage to the hamstrings using the forearm.

Another technique is to apply massage with your client supine. In this position, the hamstrings are shortened, and this can be helpful. This technique is ideal for clients who cannot lay prone because of injury; however, the technique is not appropriate for all clients, some of whom might not wish to place their leg in this position.

Ensure the client is correctly draped in a towel, if necessary. Apply gentle strokes with your forearm (figure 4.2a) or fist (figure 4.2b), gliding from just below the knee to the ischium.

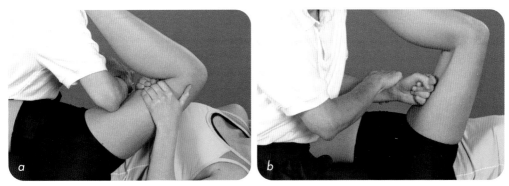

Figure 4.2   Massage to the hamstrings in the supine position using (a) the forearm or (b) the fist.

TIP

Instead of the client holding their leg, practise resting their leg on your shoulder.

Active Stretches

Active stretches are particularly useful, provided that the client remains within a pain-free range. This may mean that the client avoids lengthening the muscle at the end-of-joint range. Begin with gentle stretches, such as those shown in figures 4.3a and 4.3b, which tense the tissues not only of the calf but also of the hamstrings. Alternatively, refer to figure 5.39 in chapter 5.

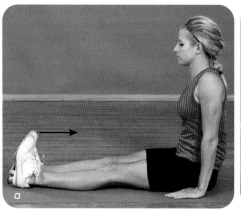 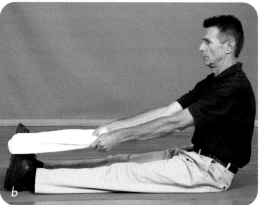

Figure 4.3 Stretching of all the tissues of the posterior lower limb, including the hamstrings, in the early stage of recovery using *(a)* active dorsiflexion or *(b)* a towel to increase tension.

Passive Stretches

Passive stretching is not recommended for hamstring strains but can be very useful when the muscle is healed, especially if adhesions have resulted in a sensation of tightness or have reduced muscle length.

Strengthening

Strengthening is an important part of hamstring strain rehabilitation. Chapter 8 provides details.

Tight Hamstrings

There are many reasons why tightness may develop in the posterior thigh. Tightness is commonly reported by runners and people regularly engaged in sports involving the lower limbs, such as tennis or rowing. Shortening of soft tissues of the posterior compartment of the thigh and knee is also likely to occur in people who remain seated for long periods of time, such as drivers, office workers or people with a sedentary lifestyle. Trigger point release, active and passive stretches and soft tissue release (STR) are all helpful in combatting tight hamstrings.

Massage

Massage feels soothing to receive and is likely to have a relaxing effect on muscles. However, it is unlikely that massage alone will be effective in alleviating tight hamstrings, and therefore, you may wish to use the additional techniques described here.

Trigger Point Release

Trigger points are found in the middle to lower portions of all three hamstring muscles – the semimembranosus, semitendinosus and biceps femoris (see figure 4.4). These triggers refer pain primarily to the back of the knee and proximal part of the posterior thigh and are perpetuated by activities such as sitting for prolonged periods with the knees flexed, as when driving or working at a desk or when immobilised in bed or a wheelchair after an injury or illness. Prolonged pressure to the back of the thigh is another perpetuating factor. You can palpate trigger points in this muscle group with your client in the prone, side-lying and even supine positions, in each case with the knee flexed.

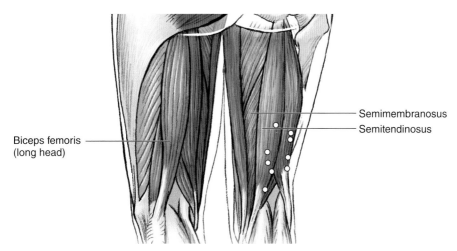

Figure 4.4   Trigger points in the hamstrings.

Studying a group of 30 physically active males with tight hamstrings and at least one trigger point, Trampas and colleagues (2010) compared the effects of trigger point release combined with stretching and of stretching alone with a control group that received no intervention. They measured knee range of motion, stretch perception, the pressure pain threshold and subjective pain (using the Visual Analogue Scale) before and after intervention. Non-painful cross-fibre friction massage was used over the trigger points in the group receiving trigger point release plus stretching. Both this group and the group receiving stretching alone showed improvements in posttreatment measures compared with the control group, and the group that received trigger point release as well as stretching showed a significant improvement in outcomes compared to the group that received stretching alone.

TIP

Pain radiating down the back of the thigh is not necessarily sciatica and can be an indication of trigger points in the hamstrings.

Use your thumb to identify trigger points (figure 4.5). You could deactivate the triggers using your thumb or apply the pressure using your elbow, with the client in a prone (figure 4.6a) or supine (figure 4.6b) position.

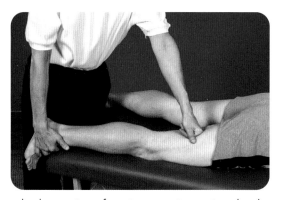

Figure 4.5 Palpating the hamstrings for trigger points using the thumb.

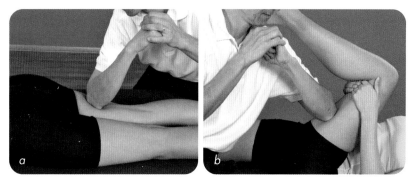

Figure 4.6 Treating trigger points using the elbow in the *(a)* prone and *(b)* supine positions.

Your client could deactivate trigger points using a tennis ball, either by sitting with the ball against a trigger point (figure 4.7a) or holding the ball against their thigh (figure 4.7b). Sitting on the ball requires less effort than holding the ball against the thigh, but care is needed because the lower limb is heavy; thus, when a client is using a ball in a seated position, they should move it approximately every 30 seconds.

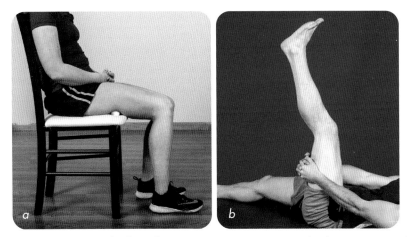

Figure 4.7 Using a tennis ball to deactivate trigger points in the hamstrings in the *(a)* sitting and *(b)* supine positions.

Stretching

There is a wide variety of stretches that are useful after deactivation of trigger points in the hamstrings, and these can all be used as standalone stretches too. Vachhani and Sharma (2021) conducted an interesting study in which they compared the effectiveness of a suboccipital muscle inhibition technique with a muscle energy technique. The position used for the Muscle Energy Technique stretch is shown in figure 4.8. You can see from the photograph that the hip is passively flexed, lengthening the hamstrings. The study participants were asked to use their leg to apply pressure to the therapist's shoulder for 7 to 10 seconds, followed by a rest of 2 to 3 seconds. The therapist then passively flexed the hip farther and held it in this new position of stretch for 30 seconds. This was repeated two more times. The rationale for use of the second technique, muscle inhibition, is that by decreasing myofascial tension in the suboccipital region, there is a decrease in tone in the knee flexors. When applying the muscle inhibition technique, the participants were supine, with the therapist cupping the base of the participant's skull such that the tips of the therapist's fingers were pressed into the participant's suboccipital muscles. This position was maintained for 2

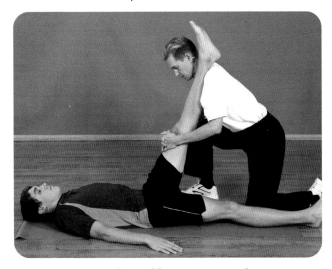

Figure 4.8 A traditional hamstring stretch.

minutes on each of 5 consecutive days. Vachhani and Sharma reported both methods to be effective in improving hamstring flexibility.

In addition to the simple stretches shown in figure 4.3, the client could use a towel, as in figure 4.9. Bear in mind that dorsiflexing the foot in this way also stretches the calf, and for some clients, this may feel uncomfortable. Clients who do not wish to do their stretches on the floor could try simply placing one leg on a stool and leaning forward to stretch the hamstrings of that limb. Obviously, this is not appropriate for clients with impaired balance. Remember that the hamstrings are hip extensors, so taking the hip into flexion, as in figure 4.10, will also help stretch these muscles. In the photograph in figure 4.10, the hamstrings of the right leg are being stretched because this is the hip that has been taken into flexion. Clients with knee problems should avoid this stretch, which places pressure on the knee opposite the thigh being stretched.

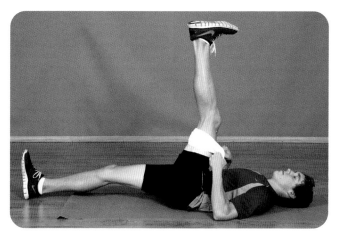

Figure 4.9 An active hamstring stretch using a towel.

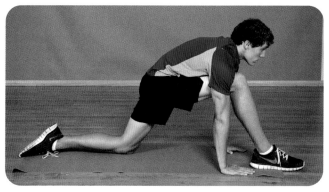

Figure 4.10 Stretching the hamstrings of the right leg.

Soft Tissue Release

There are many techniques for applying STR to the hamstrings, and these all work well for stretching this muscle group when it is perceived to be tight.

Passive Soft Tissue Release for Hamstrings: Prone

With your client in the prone position, passively shorten the hamstrings by flexing the client's knee. Lock the muscle close to its origin at the ischium (figure 4.11a) using your thumb or a soft fist. Each time you lock the fibres in this stretch, direct your pressure towards the ischium rather than perpendicularly. If using your thumb to lock the tissues, take care to press only lightly, as overuse may be damaging to your thumbs. Whilst maintaining your lock, gently stretch the muscle by extending the knee (figure 4.11b). Many clients do not feel much stretch at this point.

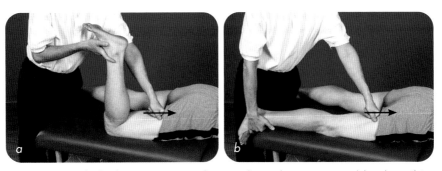

Figure 4.11 *(a)* Lock the hamstrings as close to the ischium as possible, then *(b)* stretch the tissues whilst maintaining the lock.

TIP

It is a good idea to explain to the client where the lock is going to be before beginning the treatment. Some clients may consider locking under the buttock in this way to be invasive. In figure 4.11, the therapist has chosen to place the first lock distal to the ischium, on the upper part of the thigh.

Again, with the knee passively flexed, choose a new, slightly more distal lock, perhaps in the midline of the thigh (figure 4.12a). Whilst maintaining your lock, stretch the tissues by passively extending the knee (figure 4.12b).

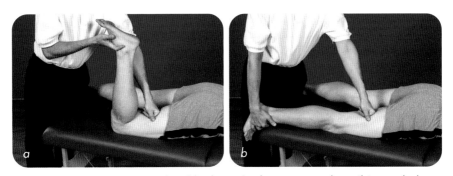

Figure 4.12 *(a)* Create a more distal lock on the hamstrings, then *(b)* stretch the tissues whilst maintaining the lock.

Work down the length of the hamstrings from proximal to distal insertions, repeating this procedure. Avoid pressing into the popliteal space behind the knee. If you are performing the technique correctly, your client will experience an increasing sensation of stretch as you work towards the hamstring tendons. If your client does not feel the stretch, you will need to do active assisted STR.

TIP

You can use STR to help assess the pliability of the hamstring muscles. Notice the resistance you feel as you work proximally to distally on these muscles. Can you sense which muscles are tightest – the biceps femoris (laterally) or the semimembranosus and semitendinosus (medially)?

If you wish to use STR to help deactivate trigger points, use your thumb to apply gentle pressure to a trigger, repeating the procedure over the trigger rather than to other parts of the muscle. Only when the trigger has dissipated should you move to another area. After STR for trigger point release, instruct your client to perform hamstring stretches to maintain length in the muscle fibres.

The hamstrings are strong, powerful muscles that require a firm lock to fix the tissues. Using a fist to lock the tissues is one method, but it is not as powerful as using a forearm (as in active assisted STR). Elbows may be used to lock the tissues, but due to the length of the lever in this case, using the elbow makes passive flexion and extension of the knee difficult and may compromise your posture as you lean forward to lock the tissues.

Active Assisted Soft Tissue Release for Hamstrings: Prone

Whilst your client is in a prone position, ask them to flex the knee. Using the side of your forearm or your elbow, lock the hamstrings close to the ischium. Direct your pressure towards the buttock to take up some of the slack in the soft tissues before the stretch (figure 4.13a). Leaning over to lock tissues could hurt your back, so take care to guard your posture. Take a wide stance and ensure that your upper body weight is supported by the client or treatment couch. With practice, this is easy. Whilst maintaining your lock, ask your client to lower the leg back to the couch (figure 4.13b). Release your lock.

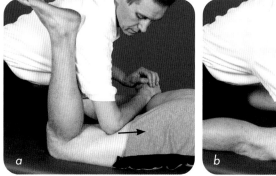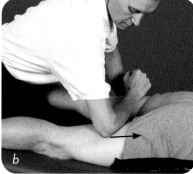

Figure 4.13 *(a)* Lock the hamstrings close to the ischium using an elbow, then *(b)* stretch the tissues as the client lowers the leg to the couch.

Choose a new lock, more distal to the first. Repeat the lock-and-stretch motion, working in lines down the posterior thigh from the ischium to the hamstring tendons. Avoid pressing into the popliteal space behind the knee.

TIP

The knee does not need to be fully flexed at the start of the technique or fully extended afterwards. Indeed, when working with a client with severe tightness on the posterior of the knee, full extension may not be desirable or possible initially.

Working on the leg closest to you (figure 4.14) is often easier than stretching across the body to the opposite leg. Using the right arm when treating the left leg (or left arm when treating the right leg) can also make application easier.

Using the point of your elbow creates a more specific lock and can be a useful alternative to thumbs when using STR to deactivate trigger points that you have first identified with finger palpation (figure 4.15). However, it is more difficult to use the elbow in this way as you reach the distal end of the muscles, where a thumb lock is better.

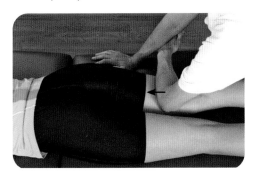 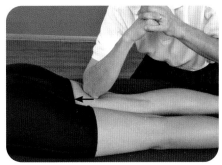

Figure 4.14 Applying soft tissue release to the leg closest to the therapist.

Figure 4.15 Using the point of the elbow to create a lock.

Active Assisted Soft Tissue Release for Hamstrings: Supine

An alternative position for applying STR to the hamstrings is to work with your client supine, their hip and knee flexed to at least 90 degrees. In this position, you can use your elbow to press into the hamstrings (figure 4.16). Maintaining pressure, ask your client to slowly extend the knee until it is straight.

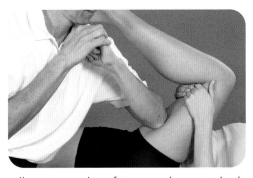

Figure 4.16 Using the elbow to apply soft tissue release to the hamstrings in the supine position.

Active Soft Tissue Release for Hamstrings

Soft tissue release can be used by your client in the seated or supine positions.

If supine, instruct your client to shorten the muscle by flexing the knee, and place a tennis ball beneath part of the hamstring muscles (figure 4.17a). Whilst holding the tennis ball, gently extend the knee (figure 4.17b).

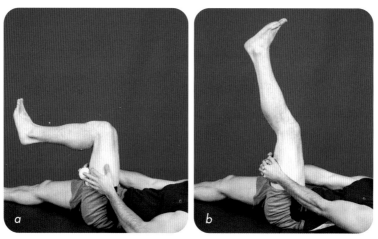

Figure 4.17 (a) Apply a ball to the hamstrings; then, maintaining the lock, (b) slowly extend the knee.

Practise this for yourself. Place your first lock (using the ball) near the ischium and gradually work down towards your knee with subsequent locks. Because the hamstrings are a large muscle group, you will need to work all over them to fully benefit from the stretches. Sometimes it is best to work systematically, perhaps starting with the biceps femoris on the lateral side of the thigh and moving from proximal to distal (ischium to knee). When you feel you have worked this section enough, move your locks to a more medial position so that you are over the semimembranosus and the semitendinosus; continue to work this area in the same way. To use the technique to deactivate trigger points in the hamstrings, palpate the muscle until you locate a trigger, place the ball over it and repeat the STR on that same spot several times until the trigger dissipates.

TIP

Observe the position of the foot and ankle of the two clients shown in figure 4.18. Most people, when they attempt active STR in the supine position, will have their foot in semi–plantar flexion (figure 4.18a). However, for even more of a stretch, the ankle may be dorsiflexed, as the client has done in figure 4.18b.

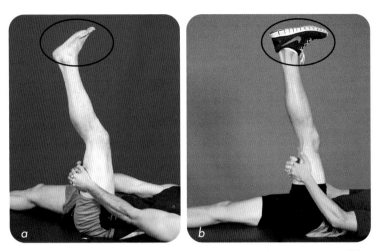

Figure 4.18 Active soft tissue release with the ankle in (a) a neutral and (b) a dorsiflexed position.

When STR is used in a seated position, start with the knee flexed and a ball between the thigh and the chair (figure 4.19a), then extend the knee (figure 4.19b). Sitting STR is useful for treating hamstrings during the day if your client has a desk job.

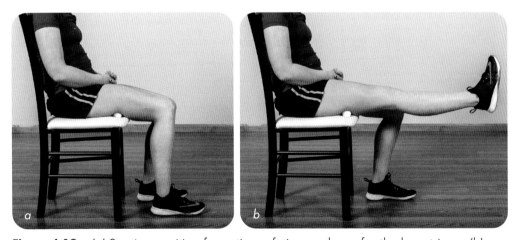

Figure 4.19 (a) Starting position for active soft tissue release for the hamstrings. (b) Extension of the knee to bring about a stretch in the tissues.

Applying STR in a seated position takes less effort than when lying down, because it does not require the ball to be held in place with the hands.

Hamstring Cramping

Involuntary contraction in the hamstrings is painful, albeit temporary. Hamstring cramping is more likely to occur after vigorous physical exertion or in patients who remain positioned for long periods of time in knee flexion. In such cases, without treatment, the cramp will eventually dissipate. However, there are other causes of cramping, and an interesting and detailed overview is provided by Swash, Czesnik and de Carvalho (2019).

Stretching

Although both active and passive stretches are helpful for hamstring cramps, active stretches may be the most beneficial, because contraction of the quadriceps or hip flexors inhibits the hamstrings, which therefore cannot contract involuntarily (i.e., cramp).

All active stretches, such as those shown in figures 4.9 and 4.10, are helpful in combatting hamstring cramps. Additionally, it is useful to teach your client how to perform an isometric contraction of their quadriceps to overcome hamstring cramping. One way to demonstrate this is to place your hand over the ankle of the leg that is cramping and ask the client to try to straighten the leg, pushing against you (figure 4.20), until the knee is extended. As with the previous stretch, contraction of the quadriceps in this way inhibits contraction of the hamstrings. Once your client understands this principle, they can use it to overcome a hamstring cramp – for example, by placing their foot under an immovable object such as a heavy bed.

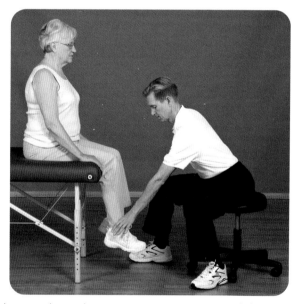

Figure 4.20   Teaching a client about isometric contraction of the quadriceps to overcome hamstring cramping.

Nocturnal leg cramps are also common in pregnancy. In a study by Anandhi, Ansari and Sivakumar (2019), 43 women reporting nocturnal lower limb cramps were divided into two groups. Group A performed non-stretching exercises (simple ankle dorsiflexion and plantar flexion) plus stretching exercises, and group B performed only the non-stretching exercises. The stretching exercises performed by group A were for the hamstrings and soleus muscles. Both groups completed their exercises three times a day for 4 weeks and were assessed before and after the intervention using the Visual Analogue Scale and a muscle and joint measurement questionnaire. The researchers found that there was a statistically significant reduction in the reported intensity of muscle cramps in the group that performed stretching exercises, leading the authors to conclude not only that stretching should be used to reduce nocturnal muscle cramps in antenatal women but that these stretches should be taught in antenatal classes as a preventative measure. If you are working with antenatal clients, it is important to remember that due to the hormone relaxin, ligaments are more lax throughout the body, so stretches should be performed slowly and carefully, avoiding straining at the end-of-joint range.

Passive stretches are also useful. The hamstrings sometimes cramp when clients are lying prone and actively flex their knees or, more commonly, when they are receiving massage in this position after a sporting event. In either case, it is useful to have some stretches to help overcome cramping.

If the cramp occurs when the client is prone, ask them to flex their knee and push their ankle into your hand (figure 4.21), contracting their quadriceps to extend their knee. Contraction of the quadriceps in this way inhibits the hamstrings and helps reduce the cramp. Ask the client to push their leg back down onto the therapy couch (or floor, if you are working on the floor) as you apply gentle resistance.

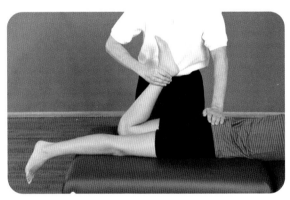

Figure 4.21 Overcoming a hamstring cramp using isometric contraction of the quadriceps.

Massage

Massage may feel soothing for the client who has experienced a hamstring cramp, but it is unlikely to be as effective as isometric contraction of the quadriceps and active or passive stretching of the hamstrings. When using massage, it is important to focus on the use of slow, deep strokes rather than techniques such as tapotement, because the goal of massage when treating a cramp is to reduce excitability in the nervous system and thereby reduce muscle tension. Tapotement is a stimulatory technique and is best avoided in the treatment of cramps.

Tight Quadriceps

The quadriceps may feel tight as a result of a sporting activity or after injury.

Massage

Once you have warmed the area using effleurage and petrissage, applying deep massage to the quadriceps is helpful to reduce feelings of tightness in this muscle group. For example, you could glide from just superior to the patella to the proximal end of the thigh using your forearm (figure 4.22a), or you could grip and squeeze the muscle (figure 4.22b).

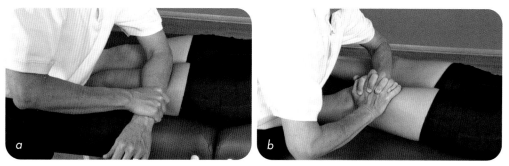

Figure 4.22 Applying deep tissue massage to the quadriceps by *(a)* gliding with the forearm or *(b)* gripping.

Trigger Point Release

Deactivation of trigger points in the thigh can also help reduce feelings of tightness. Four common trigger points are found in the quadriceps. The trigger point at the proximal attachment of the rectus femoris is close to the anterior superior iliac spine (figure 4.23) and refers pain into the knee. To identify the rectus femoris, palpate the area as you have your client perform isometric knee extension in a manner that does not engage the hip. The rectus femoris will contract, and you will be able to palpate it for this trigger.

Two trigger points in the vastus medialis (figure 4.23) refer pain to the medial thigh and knee. To palpate for these trigger points, either stand facing the side of the couch with the client in the supine position and gently glide your fingers from the adductors through to the vastus medialis or begin at the knee and palpate from the knee to the hip.

Trigger points exist in the proximal, distal and middle portions of the vastus lateralis, one of which is shown in figure 4.23. The section on iliotibial band friction syndrome in chapter 5 gives more information on how to treat the lateral thigh area.

There are trigger points in the vastus intermedialis (not shown in figure 4.23), and they refer pain over the anterolateral portion of the thigh.

The trigger points in the quadriceps are aggravated by trigger points in the hamstrings, and they may not resolve unless the hamstrings are first addressed. Tight hamstrings can prevent full knee extension, meaning that the hamstrings are unnecessarily strained during weight bearing. Trigger points in the hamstring muscles are perpetuated by immobilisation of the thigh, as is common after injury.

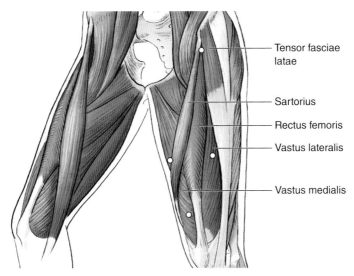

Figure 4.23 Trigger points in the quadriceps.

Espí-López and colleagues (2017) recruited 60 people with patellofemoral pain to compare the effectiveness of adding dry needling into trigger points to manual therapy and exercise. For 3 weeks, half the group received manual therapy and exercise and half the group received the same manual therapy and exercise plus dry needling into trigger points into the vastus medialis and vastus lateralis muscles. Outcome measures used were the Knee Injury and Osteoarthritis Outcome Score, the Knee Society Knee Scoring System, the International Knee Documentation Committee Subjective Knee Form, and the Numerical Pain Rating Scale. Measures were taken at baseline, 15 days posttreatment, and 3 months later. Both groups showed moderate to large improvements in all scores; no significant differences existed between the two groups, leading the authors to conclude that combining dry needling to trigger points with a manual therapy and exercise intervention did not result in improved outcomes for patients with knee pain and disability.

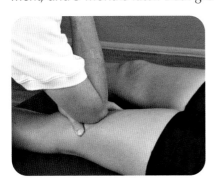

Figure 4.24 Using the elbow with care on the quadriceps.

One way to apply pressure is using your elbow. Position your hand and elbow as shown in figure 4.24, with the client's knee supported with a bolster if necessary. Using oil, apply pressure with your elbow, and use your hand to guide your elbow slowly up towards the hip. Take care that your guide hand does not encroach on the client's inner thigh.

TIP

The quadriceps can be bulky muscles, so do not be tempted to apply this technique without a guide hand, because it can be difficult to stay in place.

Alternatively, you could teach your client how to deactivate the trigger points by resting on a ball (figure 4.25). Remember to advise caution against keeping the ball in the same place for too long.

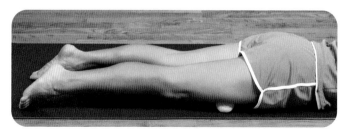

Figure 4.25   Deactivation of a trigger point in the quadriceps using a ball.

Stretching

Both active and passive stretches are helpful to alleviate the sensation of tight quadriceps and should be used after the deactivation of trigger points.

Passive Stretches

Figures 4.26*a* and 4.26*b* show common ways to passively stretch the quadriceps. If your client does not feel the stretch in this position, use of a small towel beneath the knee (figure 4.26*b*) can be helpful to extend the hip and create a deeper stretch of the rectus femoris.

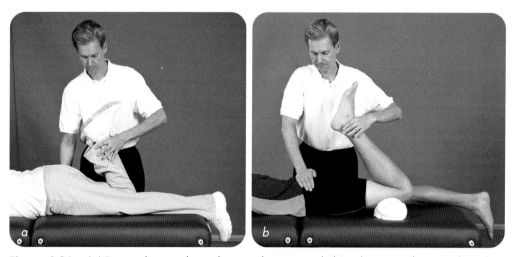

Figure 4.26   *(a)* Passively stretching the quadriceps and *(b)* enhancing the stretch with use of a towel.

Active Stretches

The quadriceps can be actively stretched in the lying (figure 4.27) or standing (figure 4.28) position. In each, the client needs to be able to reach behind their body to hold their ankle, and this requires good flexibility in the muscles of the chest and anterior shoulder joint. The standing stretch is not appropriate for clients with poor balance or who cannot bear weight through their hip, knee or ankle. To make this stretch safer, ask the client to perform it against a wall for support or to place one hand on a table for balance. The stretch in figure 4.28 could also be performed in the side-lying position.

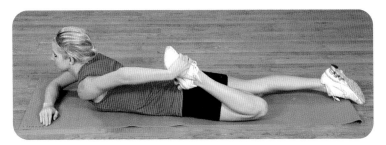

Figure 4.27　An active quadriceps stretch in the prone position.

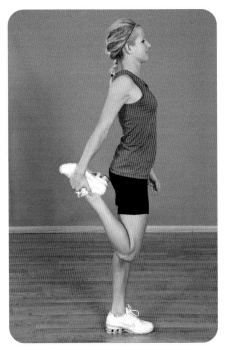

Figure 4.28　An active quadriceps stretch in the standing position.

Soft Tissue Release

Active assisted STR works well to stretch the quadriceps. One advantage of this technique is that you will be able to achieve a strong, broad lock on these powerful muscles. This method is useful if you find that a general stretching programme for the quadriceps is not targeting specific tissues. For example, by positioning a lock to the lateral side of the thigh, you are more likely to access the vastus lateralis.

With your client sitting, lock the proximal portion of the quadriceps with the client's knee in active extension, directing your pressure towards the hip (figure 4.29a). Once the knee is flexed (figure 4.29b), release your lock and repeat, placing a new lock slightly more distal to the first. Work your way down the quadriceps from hip to knee. Work slowly and carefully as you approach the distal end of the quadriceps; this increases the stretch and thus places greater pressure on the patella.

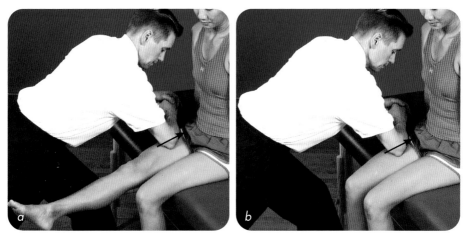

Figure 4.29 (a) Lock the quadriceps using the soft side of the elbow and (b) maintain the lock as your client flexes the knee to bring about a stretch in the quadriceps.

Note that the knee does not need to be fully flexed for the client to feel a stretch in the tissues. Practise locking the vastus lateralis and rectus femoris to locate areas of tension.

TIP

Although you can also perform this stretch using your left arm to lock the client's right quadriceps, both you and the client may find this position slightly invasive.

Active Soft Tissue Release for the Quadriceps With a Tennis Ball

Another approach is to teach your client how to apply STR to their quadriceps. This technique may be uncomfortable for some people, because the leg's entire weight is on the tennis ball. As with deactivation of trigger points, instruct your client to lie face down on a mat and position a tennis ball beneath the thigh, with the knee in extension (figure 4.30a). Then, simply have them flex the knee (figure 4.30b).

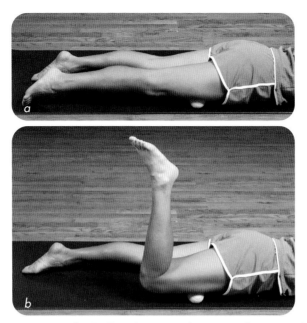

Figure 4.30 *(a)* Positioning of a ball at the start of active soft tissue release for the quadriceps followed by *(b)* active knee flexion, which brings about the stretch.

Encourage your client to practise positioning the ball against various parts of the thigh, and notice where they most feel the stretch. Position the ball near the hip at first; with subsequent locks, work towards the knee.

TIP

Pressing the pelvis forward (flattening the lumbar spine in a posterior pelvic tilt) increases the stretch in both positions.

Konrad and colleagues (2022) conducted a systematic review of the use of foam rolling to increase joint range of motion. Their review included an assessment of studies in which foam rolling was used on the quadriceps. They concluded that responses appeared to be muscle or joint specific. That is, foam rolling the quadriceps was likely to increase the range of motion in the hip and knee joints but not necessarily in other joints. Konrad and colleagues also concluded that interventions longer than 4 weeks were needed to induce gains in range of motion. Therefore, if you believe tightness in your client's quadriceps is not simply a sensation of, for example, muscle stiffness but may correspond with a shortened muscle and that lengthening this muscle to improve joint range of motion would be a valuable treatment goal, then teaching your client how to use a foam roller is likely to be helpful.

Quick Questions

1. List four ways to identify a hamstring strain.

2. When a client is using soft tissue release to their hamstrings in the supine position, what effect does changing the position of the ankle have?

3. After what duration of time should a client move a ball when using it to deactivate trigger points in the sitting position?

4. What is the effect of placing a towel beneath the knee when stretching the quadriceps in the prone position?

5. For a client who experiences tight quadriceps, what simple tool might you suggest would be helpful to use?

Knee, Calf and Shin

Learning Outcomes

After reading this chapter, you should be able to do the following:

- Explain why active stretches are more appropriate than passive stretches for acute calf muscle strain.
- Demonstrate passive stretches for calf cramps, tight calf muscles and shin splints.
- Teach active stretches for use with calf cramps, tight calf muscles and shin splints.
- Apply trigger point release to the calf and tibialis anterior and explain how to use this for the treatment of iliotibial band friction syndrome.
- Explain and give the rationale for which techniques are most appropriate when treating someone with osteoarthritis in the knee or after knee surgery.
- Demonstrate taping for genu recurvatum, genu varum and genu valgum.
- Describe the conditions presented in this chapter for which massage may be an appropriate hands-on technique and give your rationale for this.

In anatomical terms, *leg* refers to the part of the lower limb beneath the knee. This chapter discusses conditions affecting leg muscles (strain of the calf, tight calf muscles, cramp in the calf, shin splints, tight tibialis anterior and tight peroneal muscles), conditions relating specifically to the knee joint (osteoarthritis in the knee and knee surgery) and four postures relating to the knee (genu recurvatum, genu flexum, genu varum and genu valgum). Iliotibial band friction syndrome does not fit nicely into these categories because it is a condition postulated to be due to biomechanical factors plus factors affecting the fascia of the thigh, which, combined, cause knee pain.

Calf Muscle Strain

Calf muscle strains are tears in muscle fibres of the calf and may involve the gastrocnemius, soleus or both. Strains vary in severity from a few fibres being torn to complete rupture. Localised pain and swelling increase with the severity of the tear. The ability to actively plantar flex is reduced, and there is pain on stretching the calf. Scar tissue is laid down as part of the healing process, the quantity of which depends on the severity of the injury and the quality of rehabilitation the client receives. Large amounts of scar tissue may impair function. Meek and colleagues (2022) provide a nice overview of calf strain in athletes.

Massage

Massage is contraindicated in the acute stage of a calf strain. In sub-acute stages, light effleurage may help with recovery, but caution is needed to avoid damage to tissues whilst they repair. Gentle massage superior to the site of the tear could be helpful in aiding lymphatic drainage, but deep tissue massage should be avoided.

Stretching

Even where a strain is believed to be mild, all forms of stretching should be avoided in the acute stages of injury, during which time it is important to allow tissues to begin their repair process.

In the sub-acute stage, pain, swelling and inflammation have subsided. It is wise to be cautious in recommending stretches during this stage, because tissues are not yet healed and overzealous stretching could result in reinjury to the muscle, delaying the healing process.

Active Stretches

With care, active stretches may be used, provided that the client remains within a pain-free range. Dorsiflexion of the ankle in a non–weight-bearing position, either seated on a chair or with the legs extended as in figure 5.1, is a good starting stretch. Towards the end of the healing process, progression to standing calf stretches such as those shown in the section on tight calf muscles is recommended if the client believes the calf is particularly tight. Remember that with calf strains, pain subsides before healing is complete, and clients should be encouraged to stop if any of the stretches cause pain.

Passive Stretches

Passive stretching is not recommended for calf muscle strains, but it can be helpful in later stages when the calf may feel tight.

Strengthening

Please see chapter 9 for suitable calf strengthening exercises.

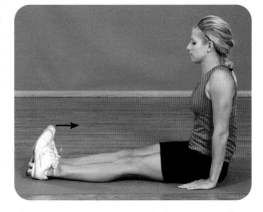

Figure 5.1 A non–weight-bearing calf stretch used in early recovery from a calf strain.

Tight Calf Muscles

Many people suffer from tight calf muscles. The muscles in the posterior compartment of the leg bring about not only plantar flexion of the foot and ankle but also flexion of the knee (gastrocnemius), inversion of the foot and ankle (tibialis anterior and posterior) and flexion of the toes (long toe flexors). It is not surprising that clients who engage in sporting activities that use the leg muscles may be prone to tension in these areas, as might people who wear high heels (which force the ankle into plantar flexion). Clients who remain seated for long periods of time may also experience shortening of tissues in this compartment, because the gastrocnemius and the fascia associated with this part of the lower limb are held in a shortened position.

Massage, trigger point release, both active and passive stretching and soft tissue release (STR) are all helpful for treating tight calves.

Massage

Although many therapists treat the calves with a client in the prone position, two useful techniques with the client supine and two with the client in a side-lying position are described here. These techniques are a nice way to treat the calf muscle in clients who cannot lay prone.

One method is to flex your client's knee and gently sit on their foot to support the limb (otherwise, they might try to keep the knee flexed rather than relaxing). Using oil, cup the distal end of the calf and squeeze it gently, allowing your palms to slide off the muscle, pulling it gently away from the bone (figure 5.2). To assist venous and lymphatic drainage, work from the ankle to the belly of the muscle just below the knee, rather than from the knee to the ankle. With the knee flexed and the ankle plantar flexed, the muscles of the posterior calf are in a passively shortened position; the gentle traction of these muscles away from the tibia feels pleasurable for most clients. However, this is a much more powerful technique than it might initially appear to be, so start gently and gradually build up the strength of your grip.

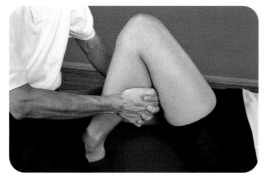

Figure 5.2   Squeezing the calf muscles away from the tibia.

Another method of treating a tight calf muscle in the supine position is to use your forearm. Flex your client's knee and gently sit on their foot to support the limb (otherwise, they might keep the knee flexed rather than relaxing). Use your forearm to

---

effleurage from the ankle to below the knee (figure 5.3). Practise pulling your forearm up and across the calf, sliding it from your elbow to your wrist as you do so. Support the client's knee with your other hand. Change forearms and repeat the procedure.

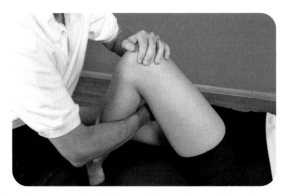

Figure 5.3 Using the forearm to 'roll' the calf muscle with the client supine.

Various deep tissue massage techniques can be used with your client in the prone position, four of which are described here. If you position your client with their feet off the end of the treatment couch so they can dorsiflex at the ankle, this will be helpful should you later wish to use STR.

The first technique is to use your forearm (figure 5.4a). Using oil, lean onto the client starting just above the Achilles tendon and glide slowly and firmly up the calf, stopping before you reach the popliteal space at the back of the knee. Notice that you can angle your forearm to redirect your pressure to the medial side of the calf using this arm, but to massage the lateral calf more firmly, you need to switch to your other arm, keeping your wrist and hand high so they do not intrude on the client's opposite leg.

As an alternative to using your forearm, try using reinforced fists. Starting where the gastrocnemius and soleus muscles insert into the Achilles tendon, press into the calf, gliding up the tissue and stopping before you reach the popliteal space at the back of the knee (figure 5.4b). Keep your elbows and wrists straight as far as possible. The therapist in figure 5.4b is using two hands. Practise what it feels like to press through a single fist, perhaps supporting your wrist with the other hand.

For even greater pressure, you could use your elbow (figure 5.4c). Locate the Achilles tendon and place your elbow against the calf, supported by the web of your thumb. Start where the gastrocnemius and soleus muscles insert into the Achilles tendon. Using oil, glide firmly and slowly up the calf, using your hand to keep your elbow from slipping off the bulk of the muscle. This technique can be used to apply compression alone to a specific spot, should this be required – for example, when deactivating trigger points in the calf.

Finally, squeezing the calf is another method of applying deep tissue massage. Start by flexing your client's knee and resting it against your shoulder, passively shortening the calf muscles. This position has the added benefit of aiding venous and lymphatic drainage from the ankle. Starting close to the Achilles tendon, squeeze the muscles away from the bone, working from the ankle towards the knee (figure 5.4d).

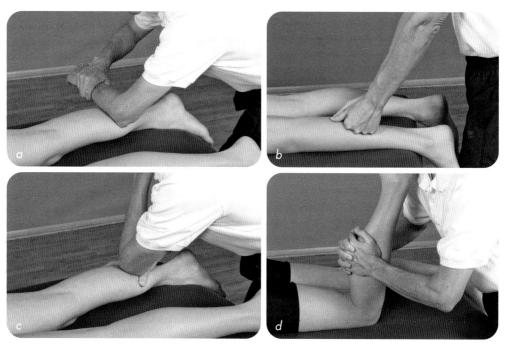

Figure 5.4 Massage tissue techniques for the calf include use of the *(a)* forearm, *(b)* fist and *(c)* elbow and *(d)* squeezing the calf.

Working with your client in a side-lying position is useful for stubbornly tight calves and when needing to treat specific areas of tightness. However, because this technique is so powerful, be cautious not to massage too deeply too soon.

Start where the calf muscles insert into the Achilles tendon. Using a reinforced fist or fists, glide firmly from this point to the medial side of the knee, compressing the tissues as you go (figure 5.5a). Once the tissues are warmed, you could work more deeply using your elbow. Touch the calf with your elbow, then glide slowly but firmly up the medial side of the calf in a continuous line (figure 5.5b).

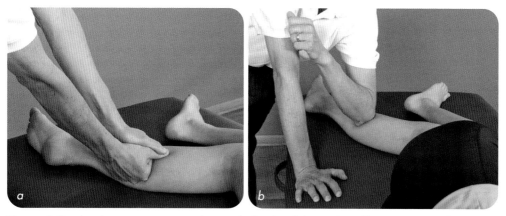

Figure 5.5 Applying massage to the medial side of the right calf using *(a)* reinforced fists or *(b)* an elbow.

Trigger Point Release

Figure 5.6 shows trigger points in the medial and lateral portions of the gastrocnemius muscle. The medial triggers refer pain primarily to the instep and medial aspect of the posterior knee, radiating on the medial aspect of the calf, whilst the lateral triggers refer pain locally and to the lateral inferior knee region. These triggers are aggravated by forceful plantar flexion of the ankle, as might occur when going *en pointe* in ballet or when walking up a steep hill. They are also perpetuated by compression of the calf, as when wearing tight socks or sitting with the legs outstretched and the calves resting on a footstool. Prolonged passive plantar flexion is also likely to aggravate triggers, as occurs when sleeping or wearing high heels.

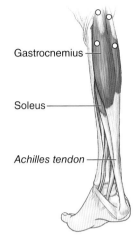

Figure 5.6 Trigger points in the calf.

Grieve, Barnett and colleagues (2013) examined myofascial trigger point therapy for the triceps surae in 10 participants with calf pain. Baseline measurements were taken before and after each treatment: the pressure pain threshold, the presence of trigger points, ankle dorsiflexion range of movement, the Lower Extremity Functional Scale and a verbal numerical rating scale. A therapist found trigger points in the gastrocnemius and soleus muscles using a thumb, then passively stretched the calf. Participants were also advised to self-treat their trigger points using a tennis ball or foam roller at least once a day, followed by active stretching of the calf. Thirteen active triggers had been identified at baseline across the 10 participants, which reduced to zero after the intervention. However, the 31 latent trigger points that had been identified across the participants were only reduced to 30. Ankle dorsiflexion for both the gastrocnemius and soleus improved after treatment, as did the pressure pain scores for all participants.

Grieve, Cranston and colleagues (2013) also explored deactivation of latent triggers in the triceps surae of 22 recreational runners. Participants ran at least twice a week and had at least one latent trigger point in either the gastrocnemius or soleus. All had restricted ankle dorsiflexion. Trigger point release was performed with thumb pressure for 10 minutes, followed by stretching the gastrocnemius and soleus muscles for 10 seconds each. The control group received no intervention, but both groups had pretest and posttest ankle dorsiflexion measurements taken using a goniometre. Ankle dorsiflexion increased in both groups but was greater in the intervention group. In the intervention group, the increase was statistically significant compared to baseline measurements for both the soleus and gastrocnemius, leading the authors to conclude that myofascial trigger point release provided an immediate improvement in ankle dorsiflexion.

More recently, in a study involving 50 participants, Wilke, Vogt and Banzer (2018) compared the effectiveness of self–myofascial release of trigger points in the calf. They found that static pressure applied to the trigger with a foam roller was more effective at reducing the trigger than using the foam roller to slowly compress the length of the calf.

TIP

If a client complains of waking at night with a cramp in the calf, in the absence of any serious pathology, consider the presence of trigger points in the gastrocnemius.

Trigger points in the calf can be deactivated using simple elbow pressure (figure 5.7). Note that the client in the figure has been deliberately positioned with their feet off the edge of the couch because this is the position needed for STR. If you use this position to deactivate trigger points and you intend to also use STR, it will prevent your client from having to shuffle down the couch between use of these two techniques during a treatment. You could also teach your client how to deactivate triggers by resting their leg on a tennis ball (figure 5.8).

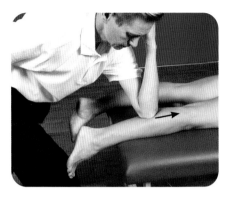

Figure 5.7   Deactivating trigger points using the elbow to apply pressure.

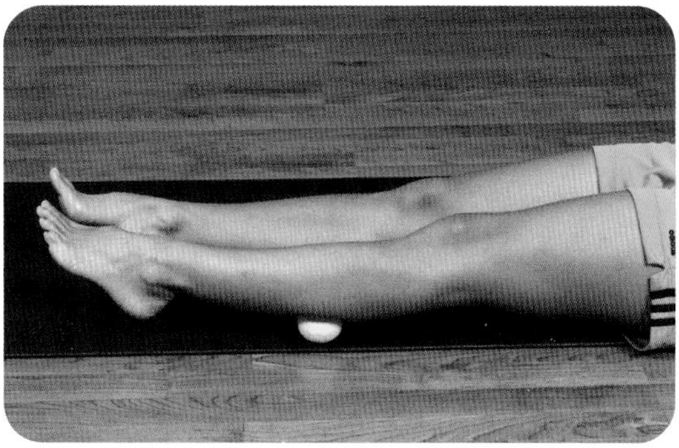

Figure 5.8   Active trigger point release.

Stretching

After trigger point release, stretch the muscle using either passive or active stretches. Stretching is a helpful stand-alone technique for relieving feelings of tightness in the calf, and a variety of options are described here.

Passive Stretches

Useful passive stretches are shown in figures 5.9a and 5.9b. In the prone position, flexing the knee focuses the stretch more to the soleus, whereas with the knee in neutral, both the gastrocnemius and soleus are stretched, as well as other ankle plantar flexors. Notice that in figure 5.9a, the therapist is using the thigh to increase dorsiflexion at the ankle, an action that requires considerable force when using your hand. The stretch shown in figure 5.9b increases the stretch to the soleus muscle but may not be appropriate for clients who are unable to lie prone or for those who have knee problems on the side being stretched (as you can see, this particular stretch puts quite a lot of pressure on the knee). Another stretch that may be helpful is to passively dorsiflex the ankle in the supine position (figure 5.9c). However, these stretches can be less effective for strong, physically active people, because the force required to promote the stretch is more difficult to apply with the client in the prone position.

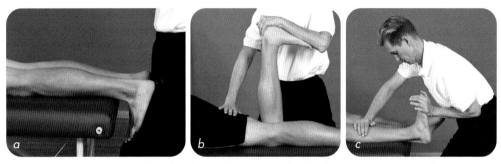

Figure 5.9 Passive stretches for the calf *(a)* using the thigh to increase dorsiflexion, *(b)* targeting the soleus muscle and *(c)* in the supine position.

Active Stretches

It could be argued that active stretches are more effective at combatting tightness than passive stretches because the client is able to use their body weight to facilitate the stretch. Simple and effective calf stretches that use the client's body weight include the standing calf stretches shown in figures 5.10*a* and 5.10*b*. Figure 5.10*a* is a traditional calf stretch (in this example, for the left leg). If your client requires a more powerful stretch, they can raise the toes, because this increases dorsiflexion. One way to do this is to place a small block beneath the toes (figure 5.10*b*).

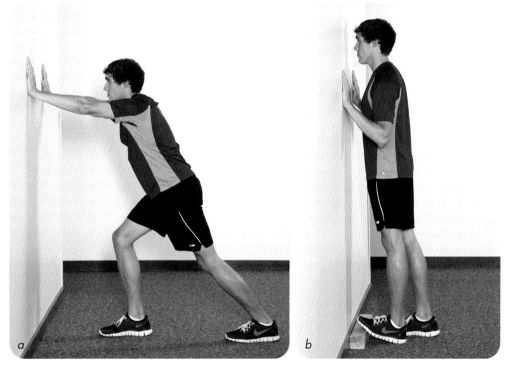

Figure 5.10 Active stretches in a standing position include *(a)* a traditional calf stretch, shown here for the left leg, and *(b)* the use of a small block to increase dorsiflexion and therefore increase the stretch.

In the first stretch (figure 5.10*a*), it is important that the client's feet are facing forwards. Try this for yourself and notice that turning the foot out slightly decreases the sensation of the stretch.

Soft Tissue Release

Soft tissue release is an excellent method to help reduce the sensation of tightness in the calf muscles, and there are many different ways to apply the lock, including gripping the calf or using the thumbs, fists, forearm or elbow.

Active Assisted Soft Tissue Release for the Calf Using Grip Lock

Perhaps one of the simplest ways to apply STR to the calf is with your client in the prone position. Passive flexion of the knee facilitates slackening of the calf muscle, which permits a deeper lock and a different stretch sensation for the client. This provides a general stretch that is not localised to a specific part of the calf.

Passively flex the client's knee and grasp the calf (figure 5.11). Whilst in this position, ask your client to plantar flex and dorsiflex the foot and ankle as you maintain the lock. Take care not to grip the muscle too hard.

When using STR in the prone position, it is first important to position your client cor-

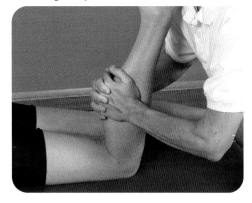

Figure 5.11 Using a grip lock on the calf.

rectly and check that you can dorsiflex their foot passively. Usually, it is best to shorten a muscle slightly before performing STR. The calf is an exception to this rule, because the foot and ankle naturally fall into plantar flexion, in which the muscles are already neutral (neither stretched nor contracted). Position your client prone with the feet off the end of the treatment couch (figure 5.12*a*). Check for clips on the edge of the treatment couch that may press into the client's foot. Make sure the client can dorsiflex at the ankle. One way to do so is to gently push the ankle into dorsiflexion (figure 5.12*b*).

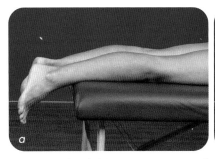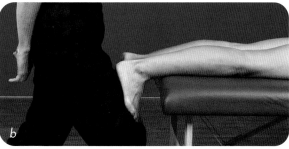

Figure 5.12 *(a)* Positioning your client on the couch and *(b)* passively dorsiflexing the ankle.

Practise positioning your thigh on various aspects of your client's foot, either medially or laterally. Find the position that provides the client with the greatest stretch. When you apply this technique, you will need to provide passive dorsiflexion of the ankle to at least 90 degrees. Notice that to do so, you need to angle the client's foot so as to stretch the calf muscle, not simply press on the foot, thereby pushing the client up the treatment table.

Passive Soft Tissue Release for the Calf Using Thumbs: Prone

Using reinforced thumbs to apply STR is useful because it is a good way to use STR to treat trigger points in the upper part of the gastrocnemius. However, it is essential for all therapists to protect their own limbs, and overuse of the thumbs should be avoided. Because they are plantar flexors, calf muscles are exceptionally strong, and it may be necessary to use a particularly firm lock when treating them. Although it may be tempting to press harder with your thumbs, you should avoid doing it.

When applying STR to the calf, it does not matter whether you start STR in the centre of the calf or to the lateral or medial side. Usually, STR applied approximately three times to one group of muscle fibres is adequate to help stretch these fibres and increase the range of motion at a joint.

Whilst standing at the end of the couch, lock the calf using reinforced thumbs, just distal to the knee joint, perhaps in the centre of the calf. Each time you lock the fibres in this stretch, direct your pressure towards the knee rather than perpendicularly (figure 5.13a). Whilst maintaining your lock, use your thigh to dorsiflex the client's ankle (figure 5.13b).

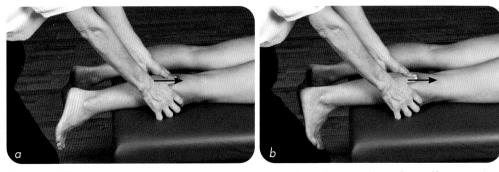

Figure 5.13 (a) Locking the calf using the thumbs, then (b) stretching the calf passively by dorsiflexing the ankle using the thigh.

Once you have dorsiflexed the ankle, release your lock, remove your thigh and move to a new locking position distal to your first lock (figure 5.14a). Dorsiflex the ankle once again (figure 5.14b).

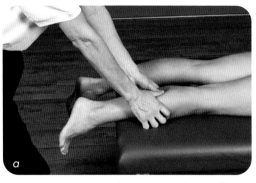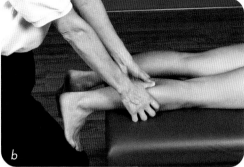

Figure 5.14 *(a)* Lock tissues in the midline of the calf, then *(b)* passively dorsiflex the ankle to bring about a stretch whilst maintaining a lock.

Once you have dorsiflexed the ankle, release the lock and your thigh. Then, place a new, more distal lock (figure 5.15*a*). Once again, passively dorsiflex the ankle (figure 5.15*b*).

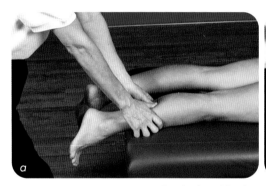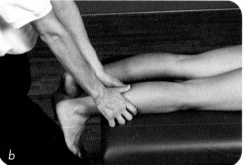

Figure 5.15 *(a)* Create a final, distal lock on the calf, then *(b)* passively stretch the calf whilst maintaining a distal lock.

Work down the length of the muscle proximally to the junction of the muscle with the Achilles tendon. Repeat this action along the same line of the calf up to three times.

TIP

The gastrocnemius, the most superficial calf muscle, is a bipennate muscle: It has two bellies. Once you have performed STR down the centre of the muscle, move to the lateral or medial aspect of the calf, following the same steps. Working on the lateral and medial sides of the calf will help you to identify trigger points here. Notice that many clients have a palpable band of tension running down their lateral calf. Could this band be thickened fascia between the lateral and posterior compartments of the leg?

Passive Soft Tissue Release for the Calf Using Fists: Prone

The only difference between applying passive STR to the calf using the fists instead of the thumbs is in the method of locking. With your client in the prone position, instead of using your thumbs, make a gentle fist to create the lock (figure 5.16*a*). Whilst maintaining your lock, gently dorsiflex the ankle (figure 5.16*b*).

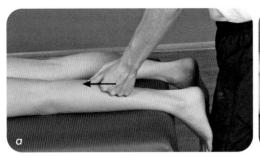 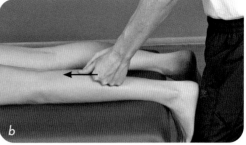

Figure 5.16 *(a)* Lock the calf using your fists, then *(b)* use your thigh to passively dorsiflex the ankle to bring about the stretch.

Passive Soft Tissue Release for the Calf Using Fists to Glide: Prone With Knee Extension

This can be a soothing form of STR for clients with large, bulky muscles for whom you find it difficult to maintain a lock or for clients with tender calves for whom a specific lock is uncomfortable.

Apply a small amount of massage medium, such as oil or wax. As you dorsiflex the ankle, use your fist to apply pressure as you glide from the ankle to the top of the calf, reducing pressure when you reach the knee (figure 5.17).

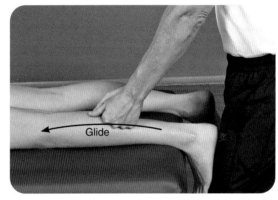

Figure 5.17 Applying gliding soft tissue release on the calf using the fists.

Passive Soft Tissue Release for the Calf Using Forearms to Glide: Prone With Knee Flexion

This method can feel soothing and also aid blood and lymph flow towards the knee. However, it can take practice to become proficient in passive dorsiflexion of the ankle with simultaneous gliding.

Rest your client's ankle on your thigh as they lie in the prone position, and place your hand on their toes (figure 5.18*a*). Using your forearm, glide from the ankle to the knee as you passively dorsiflex the ankle (figure 5.18*b*).

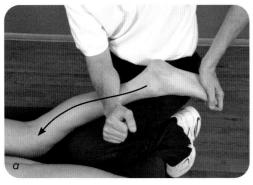
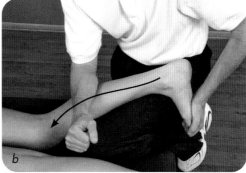

Figure 5.18 *(a)* Place your hands on the client's toes in preparation to glide up the calf, then *(b)* passively dorsiflex the ankle whilst gliding up the calf with the forearm.

Active Assisted Soft Tissue Release for the Calf Using the Elbow: Prone

Active assisted STR is helpful because the client is likely to dorsiflex to a greater extent than through passive STR to the calf and may therefore experience a greater stretch. Using the elbow is also an effective method of using STR to deactivate trigger points in addition to being a useful method of stretching the calf.

Lock the calf muscle using your elbow. Place your first lock just inferior to the knee joint, taking care not to press into the popliteal space at the back of the knee (figure 5.19*a*). Notice that the muscle naturally falls into a neutral position with the client prone and therefore does not need to be actively shortened. Whilst maintaining your lock, ask your client to pull up the toes, thus dorsiflexing the foot and ankle (figure 5.19*b*). Once the client has done so, remove your lock and move to a new position. Repeat the action. Work down the calf towards the ankle, stopping when you reach the Achilles tendon. Repeat in lines from the proximal to the distal ends of the muscle. Because constant dorsiflexion fatigues the tibialis anterior muscle, limit the time you spend on active assisted STR to the calf.

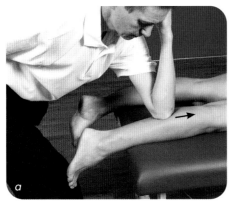
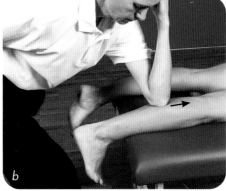

Figure 5.19 *(a)* Gentle locking of the calf using the elbow followed by *(b)* active contraction of the tibialis anterior, which brings about the stretch.

TIP

For an alternative to using your elbow, use your thumbs (figure 5.20a). For a broader lock, use your forearm (figure 5.20b).

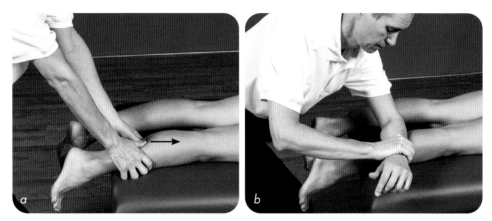

Figure 5.20   Alternative locks used for the application of active assisted soft tissue release to the calf include (a) reinforced thumbs and (b) the forearm.

Active Soft Tissue Release for the Calf: Supine

If you wish to teach your clients how to use STR to stretch their calves, show them how to place the calf on a ball (figure 5.21a). To shorten the calf, you would normally plantar flex. However, you will find that the ankle falls naturally into plantar flexion in this position. Gently dorsiflex the ankle (figure 5.21b).

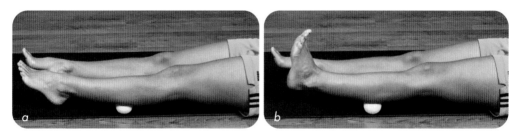

Figure 5.21   Active soft tissue release applied to the calf involves (a) positioning a ball and then (b) dorsiflexing the ankle.

TIP

For a broader, less specific lock, an alternative is to place the leg on a cylinder, such as a can, and apply the stretch.

Strengthening

Strengthening of the tibialis anterior muscle can be a useful way to reduce tightness in the calf, because the tibialis is the antagonist muscle to the gastrocnemius and soleus. Please see chapter 9 for examples of exercises.

Calf Cramping

A cramp is an involuntary contraction and is commonly felt in muscles of the calf; the exact cause is unknown. It is painful, aggravated by active or passive shortening of a muscle and often experienced at night when the ankle naturally falls into a position of plantar flexion. Of short duration, cramping subsides naturally but is nevertheless painful and limits function. Swash, Czesnik and de Carvalho (2019) provide a useful review of the pathophysiology of cramping and current treatment interventions.

Stretching

Both active and passive stretching of the calf can be helpful in reducing cramping. Remember the long toe flexors originate in the posterior calf, so stretching the toes into extension can also be helpful. See the section on stiff feet and ankles in chapter 6 for more details.

Active Stretches

Many people who experience calf cramps know that by standing up and walking about, the cramp eventually subsides. During walking, the foot is dorsiflexed, thus stretching the calf muscles. A useful way to combat a cramp is to contract the opposing muscle group, actively dorsiflexing the foot and ankle as in figure 5.22 to inhibit contraction in the muscles of the calf. The client should sustain this dorsiflexion until the cramp subsides.

However, it can be challenging to dorsiflex the ankle through its entire range of motion, so using a stretch such as in figure 5.23 may be necessary.

Calf cramping, especially at night, is common during pregnancy. The study by Anandhi, Ansari and Sivakumar (2019) described in chapter 4 concluded that stretching should be used to reduce nocturnal muscle cramps in antenatal women. An active, standing calf stretch was used in that study (figure 5.23).

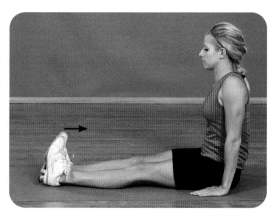

Figure 5.22   Active contraction of the ankle dorsiflexor muscles to overcome a cramp in the calf.

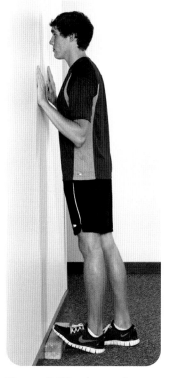

Figure 5.23   A standing stretch to overcome a cramp in the calf.

Passive Stretches

Passive stretches are useful if a cramp occurs during a massage treatment or if you happen to be treating a client before or after a sporting event. If the client is in the prone position, you could use the stretches shown in figures 5.24a and 5.24b. If the client is in the supine position, use the stretch shown in figure 5.24c.

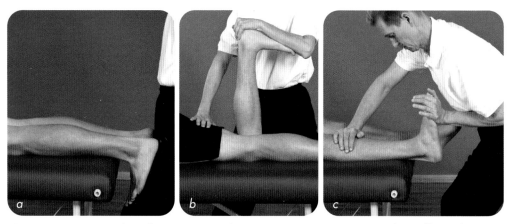

Figure 5.24 Examples of passive stretches to overcome a cramp in the calf can be applied in the (a, b) prone and (c) supine positions.

Massage

Massage alone is unlikely to reduce cramping in the calf. When using massage, it is important to focus on slow, deep strokes (a stimulatory technique) rather than techniques such as tapotement, because the goal of massage is to reduce muscle tension by reducing excitability in the nervous system.

Strengthening

Contraction of the antagonist muscle to the muscle that is cramping can be an effective way to overcome the cramp. If the cramp is in the posterior compartment of the calf (gastrocnemius and soleus), then it is important to contract the tibialis anterior, but if the cramp is in the lateral compartment (fibular muscles), then it is important to contract the invertors. Chapter 9 explains how to do this.

Shin Splints

Shin splints is a generic lay term used to describe pain on the anterior leg, commonly the result of overuse activities such as running. The therapeutic name is *medial tibial stress syndrome*. There is pain on the medial tibial border, and often, there is pes planus foot posture. The client may have a tight Achilles tendon, and dorsiflexion is usually restricted. Many factors may contribute to the development of this condition. Massage and stretching can be soothing.

Massage

Passively flex your client's knee. Starting at the ankle, use your fist to massage from the ankle to the knee (figure 5.25).

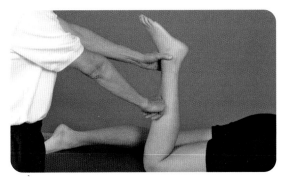

Figure 5.25   Gentle massage to the shin using a fist.

Soft Tissue Release

Soft tissue release is helpful in addressing tension in the tissues of the anterior leg and may be performed with the client in the prone or supine position.

Active Assisted Gliding Soft Tissue Release for the Tibialis Anterior: Prone

With your client in the prone position, apply a small amount of a massage medium, such as oil or wax, to the front of the leg. Starting at the ankle, gently glide your fist along the length of the tibialis anterior muscle as your client actively dorsiflexes and plantar flexes the ankle (figure 5.26).

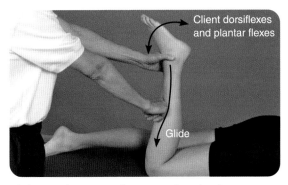

Figure 5.26   Using gliding soft tissue release on the tibialis anterior.

135

Active Assisted Soft Tissue Release for the Tibialis Anterior: Supine

To apply STR in the supine position, start by shortening the muscle. Next, apply gentle pressure to the muscle (figure 5.27a), close to its origin. Maintaining this pressure, lengthen the muscle in question by either passively or actively plantar flexing the ankle (figure 5.27b). When you have done this, select a different spot on the muscle, perhaps distal to where you first applied pressure, and repeat the process of first shortening the muscle, then applying pressure and maintaining this pressure whilst plantar flexing the ankle.

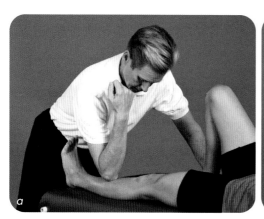 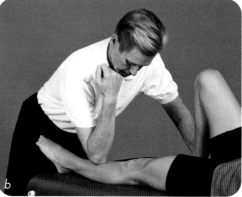

Figure 5.27 Applying active assisted soft tissue release to the tibialis anterior involves *(a)* first applying a lock with the ankle in dorsiflexion and then *(b)* asking your client to plantar flex the foot and ankle.

Note that in this example, a therapist experienced in the use of STR is using the elbow to gently compress the tibialis anterior. If you are unfamiliar with this technique, it is better to start by gently fixing or locking the muscle using your thumbs to avoid potentially bruising the tissues covering the shin.

TIP

It is obviously important to ensure that pain on the anterior shin is not the result of stress fractures, in which case, this technique would be contraindicated.

Stretching

Stretching is important following soft tissue release to the tibialis anterior. When treating someone for shin splints, stretching the calf muscles is also needed because of the likely restriction in this muscle group. Please see the previous sections on tight calf muscles and calf cramping.

Passive Stretches

Passive stretching of the tibialis anterior is not particularly effective, because this compresses the posterior ankle, squashing the Achilles tendon, and can be uncomfortable. However, adding slight traction as you perform the stretch can help reduce this compression and make the stretch feel more comfortable (figure 5.28).

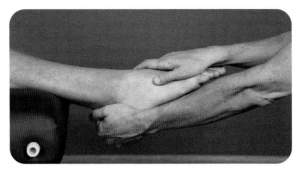

Figure 5.28   Passively stretching the tibialis anterior by plantar flexing the ankle.

Active Stretches

A simple active stretch is to point the toes, thus plantar flexing the foot and stretching the tibialis anterior (as in figure 5.29).

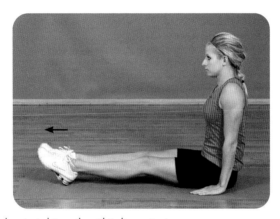

Figure 5.29   Actively stretching the tibialis anterior.

Strengthening

Strengthening of both the tibialis anterior and posterior calf muscles is crucial to recovery from shin splints, especially if your client is engaged in sporting activity or recreational fitness. Please see chapter 9 for more details.

Running Footwear and Gait

A review of the footwear the person uses when engaged in impact sports such as running is likely to be helpful, because adequate shock absorption could reduce the likelihood of reinjury. In some cases, orthotics may be useful. Use of compression stockings has also been reported to ease symptoms. If your client is a runner, referral to a specialist for analysis of their running gait could help identify whether running retraining is needed.

Tight Tibialis Anterior

When a client reports having a tight tibialis anterior, deeper techniques may be used than those for shin splints. Not only is massage helpful, but so is the deactivation of trigger points, followed by stretching, such as STR.

Massage

Once you have warmed the muscle, perhaps using techniques such as the one shown in figure 5.25, you are ready to work more deeply and perhaps more specifically on the muscle. This might be with your elbow or knuckle. Help your client get comfortable in a side-lying position. Locate the tibialis anterior by asking your client to dorsiflex the foot and ankle. Then, using your elbow (figure 5.30) or a knuckle, press gently into the muscle just above the ankle and glide slowly towards the origin. The shin is a sensitive area for most clients, so little pressure is needed when using the elbow.

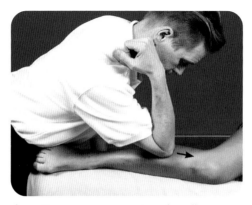

Figure 5.30   Applying deep tissue massage using the elbow.

TIP

By placing the client's foot over the end of the treatment couch, it is possible to passively turn the foot gently into inversion whilst applying this massage technique; this serves to stretch the fascia of the lateral and anterolateral leg. (Gently plantar flexing the client's ankle helps stretch the tibialis anterior.)

Trigger Point Release

A trigger point is found in the upper third of the tibialis anterior (figure 5.31) and refers pain to the dorsal aspect of the big toe and the front of the ankle. The point is easy to identify, just lateral to the ridge of the tibia. Trigger points in the tibialis anterior are likely activated by trauma to the ankle or foot. Trigger points can be deactivated by applying static pressure using the elbow (figure 5.32a), a knuckle (figure 5.32b) or a thumb.

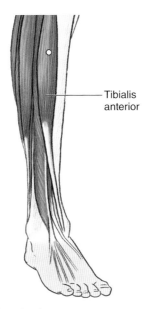

Tibialis
anterior

Figure 5.31 Trigger point in the tibialis anterior.

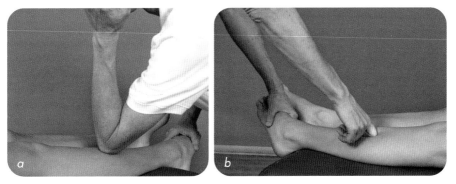

Figure 5.32 Applying static pressure using (a) the elbow or (b) a knuckle to deactivate trigger points in the tibialis anterior.

Soft Tissue Release

Although active soft tissue release to the tibialis anterior is possible using a therapy ball, it is somewhat difficult. Active assisted STR can be included as part of a massage routine where the gliding STR technique described here can be particularly helpful.

Active Assisted Soft Tissue Release for the Tibialis Anterior

There are several positions in which you could apply this technique. One of the easiest is with your client in the prone position. Ask them to dorsiflex and plantar flex their foot as you slowly glide your fist from the ankle to the knee (figure 5.33).

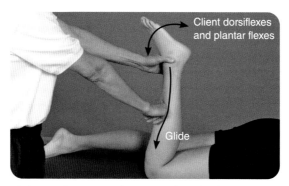

Client dorsiflexes and plantar flexes

Glide

Figure 5.33   Using gliding soft tissue release on the tibialis anterior.

For deeper pressure, position your client either side-lying or supine. Locate the tibialis anterior by asking your client to pull up the toes. Whilst the client's ankle is in dorsiflexion, lock the muscle. The tibialis anterior is a straplike muscle, and locking it gently using the elbow works well, directing your pressure towards the knee. Whilst maintaining your lock, ask your client to point the toes. Once the toes are pointed, release your lock and choose a new position, slightly more distal, for your second lock. With the ankle in dorsiflexion, lock in and repeat, working proximally to distally as long as the client feels the stretch and it is comfortable.

TIP

The tibialis anterior becomes tendinous fairly quickly, so it is not necessary to work all the way down the length of the muscle to the ankle; to do so may be uncomfortable for the client because this muscle lies over the tibia.

Strengthening

Strengthening the muscles of the posterior calf can help reduce feelings of tightness in the tibialis anterior. Please see chapter 9 for more information.

Tight Peroneal (Fibular) Muscles

The peroneal (fibular) muscles of the lateral leg are primarily evertors of the foot and ankle. They can become shortened in people who are flatfooted, and these muscles are prone to cramping in some people. Unfortunately, they are difficult to stretch actively or passively, because this requires inversion of the ankle, and a client can still report feelings of tightness even with full inversion. Massage can be soothing but is unlikely to have a lasting effect on sensations of tightness. One of the best methods to treat these muscles is STR, because it can be localised to trigger points to release them and reduce sensations of tightness.

Trigger points in the peroneal (fibular) muscles refer pain to the lateral malleolus, to the anterolateral aspect of the ankle and sometimes to the heel (figure 5.34). You can easily locate them by palpating the lateral side of the leg with your client in a side-lying position. Take care when palpating the proximal end of the muscle, because the common peroneal nerve courses around the head of the fibula here, and pressure to the nerve causes a tingling sensation.

Immobilisation of the ankle for any reason may perpetuate triggers, and clients with triggers may report frequent ankle sprains or a feeling that the ankle is unstable. Other perpetuating factors include leg-length discrepancy, flatfootedness, wearing high heels and prolonged plantar flexion.

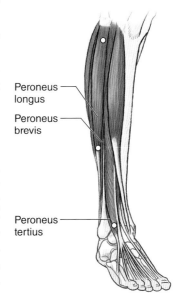

Peroneus longus

Peroneus brevis

Peroneus tertius

In a randomised controlled trial, Rossi and colleagues (2017) examined whether spinal and peripheral dry needling were any better than peripheral dry needling for people with a history of lateral ankle sprain. Twenty participants with a history of ankle sprain were randomly assigned to one of two groups. One group received dry needling into trigger points in the multifidus and fibular muscles; the other group received dry needling to fibular muscles alone. Measurements were taken at baseline, immediately after the intervention and 6 or 7 days later. Measurements included the Foot and Ankle Disability Index, the Cumberland Ankle Instability Tool, unilateral strength, performance on a balance and hop test and pain measured on the Visual Analogue Scale. There was no significant difference between the groups at the end of the study, leading the authors to conclude that dry needling of the multifidus in addition to dry needling of trigger points in the fibular muscles did not result in short-term improvements over and above dry needling trigger points in the fibular muscles alone.

Figure 5.34 Trigger points in the peroneal (fibular) muscles.

Soft Tissue Release

With your client in the side-lying position, ask them to evert the foot; demonstrate what you mean. Lock the muscle, which is now in a shortened position, directing your pressure towards the knee (figure 5.35a). For demonstration purposes, the therapist in the photo has chosen to use reinforced thumbs to lock the muscle and has positioned the client's leg on a bolster to facilitate movement of the ankle. Alternatively, you can use your elbow, using caution to prevent bruising the tissue against the fibula. Whilst maintaining your lock, ask the client to invert the foot. You may want to show the client how to do this motion first, and rather than using the term *inversion*, ask them to turn the sole of the foot inwards (figure 5.35*b*). Work in a single line down the muscle, from proximal to distal, as long as the client feels the stretch and remains comfortable.

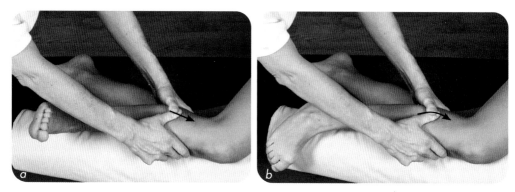

Figure 5.35   Maintaining a lock on the peroneal (fibular) muscles using *(a)* reinforced thumbs followed by *(b)* active inversion of the ankle produces a stretch in these muscles.

Strengthening

Tension in the fibular muscles can be reduced by strengthening the invertors of the ankle. Chapter 9 provides details.

Podiatry

If your client overpronates their foot, referral to a podiatrist could be useful in identifying whether the use of orthotics would help the incidence of fibular tightness or cramping.

Osteoarthritis in the Knee

Osteoarthritis is a natural part of the aging process and is caused by degeneration of the hyaline cartilage of synovial joints. It commonly occurs in older adults in weight-bearing joints such as the hips, knees and lumbar spine. As the condition worsens, there is increasing pain, swelling and inflammation of the joint as more and more of the hyaline cartilage wears away. Degeneration of the hyaline cartilage covering the articulating bones of the knee joint is painful when the patient stands and during weight-bearing activities such as climbing or descending stairs, when the articulating surfaces of the knee joint grind together. In advanced stages of the condition, the knee becomes less stable.

When describing this condition to your client, it is extremely important to explain that osteoarthritis is a natural part of the aging process and that someone can have osteoarthritis and be symptom free. Hearing terms such as *wear and tear*, *degenerating* or *chronic* can make a person fearful, and this can be a barrier to management of the condition. Therefore, the words you use when treating clients with this condition need to be chosen carefully.

Guidelines from the National Institute for Health and Care Excellence (NICE) (2022) recommend providing only soft tissue techniques alongside therapeutic exercise, because there is not enough evidence to support the use of manual therapy alone.

Trigger Point Release

Researchers Lin and colleagues (2022) examined nine randomised controlled trials relating to the treatment of knee pain to evaluate the effectiveness of acupuncture inactivation of myofascial trigger points in people with knee osteoarthritis. The studies they examined included a total of 724 patients. Lin and colleagues concluded that acupuncture inactivation of the triggers was a safe, effective and rapid intervention for the treatment of knee osteoarthritis.

Massage

Massaging is useful for pain management in clients with osteoarthritis but is unlikely to affect the underlying condition. As the condition progresses and weight bearing through the knee becomes increasingly painful, it is common for someone with osteoarthritis to start bearing more weight through their opposite leg, and they may begin to experience pain and dysfunction in that leg too. Massaging the quadriceps and hamstrings is useful for soothing postexercise tension.

Stretching

Gentle stretching of the hamstrings and quadriceps is helpful for alleviating tension, although it is necessary to avoid pressure through the knee. Often, the joint is swollen and painful to move. Whilst stretching is not a treatment per se for osteoarthritis in the knee, the movement required to perform some of the stretches helps increase synovial fluid in the joint and helps combat the muscular tension that may develop in patients enrolled in a lower limb strengthening programme before knee surgery for this particular condition.

Active Stretches

Ask your client to gently bend and straighten the leg whilst in the supine position, flexing and extending the knee as shown in figure 5.36. Flexion helps stretch the quadriceps, whilst extension tenses the popliteus, the hamstrings, the heads of the gastrocnemius and the fascia associated with these muscles. This is the most simple stretch for knee osteoarthritis and is helpful for clients who are limited in their mobility and ability to perform other stretches.

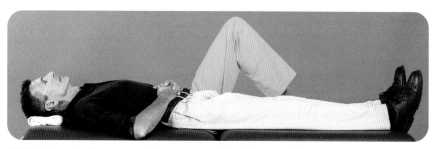

Figure 5.36   Simple flexion and extension of the knee in the supine position for clients who have severe mobility limitations.

Passive Stretches

You could start by assisting your client in knee flexion and extension in the supine position as shown in figure 5.36. You can gently add pressure in the position of flexion, provided that this does not elicit pain. Alternatively, gentle traction to the lower limb helps stretch all lower limb tissues, including those of the knee joint, and may provide temporary relief. To do this, gently cup the client's ankle and apply slow, steady traction, one limb at a time, as shown in figure 5.37. Obviously, this also tractions the ankle and hip joints and cannot be performed if there are any acute conditions affecting either of these. Experiment to discover the handhold that works best for you.

   If your client is able to lie in the prone position, you could gently stretch the quadriceps as in figure 5.38.

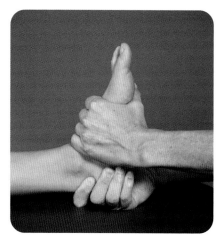

Figure 5.37   Handhold used to apply gentle passive traction to the lower limb, including the knee joint.

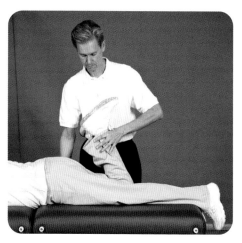

Figure 5.38   Gentle passive knee flexion in the prone position.

Strengthening

The Osteoarthritis Research Society International (Bannuru et al. 2019) report that core treatments deemed safe for most individuals with osteoarthritis in the knee are structured, land-based programmes and mind–body programmes such as tai chi and yoga. They state that aquatic exercise demonstrates robust evidence for pain management and objective measurements for function. People with osteoarthritis in the knee are usually advised to take part in exercises designed to strengthen the quadriceps and hamstrings, with the goal of providing additional muscular support to the joint. Please refer to chapter 8 for information about specific exercises that might be of benefit.

Bracing and Walking Aids

In their literature review of conservative treatment for knee osteoarthritis, Lim and Al-Dadah (2022) reported that clinical studies do not support the use of braces: They are ineffective at improving overall pain or function, and there is often non-compliance due to skin chafing. The Osteoarthritis Research Society International (Bannuru et al. 2019) specifically recommend against the use of knee bracing. According to the evidence-based guidelines provided by NICE (2022), bracing should not be routinely provided for people with knee osteoarthritis except where there is atypical biomechanical loading and joint instability, and therapeutic exercise is ineffective without the addition of an aid or device; however, the addition of an aid or device is likely to improve function. The NICE do, however, recommend considering the use of walking aids for people with lower limb osteoarthritis.

After Knee Surgery

Patients who have undergone surgery to the knee for conditions such as total or partial knee replacement, repair of cruciate ligaments or removal of a meniscus usually experience considerable swelling in the joint, which may have been immobilised after the operation. It is therefore not uncommon for such patients to experience stiffness in the knee and a decreased range of motion post-operatively. Massage and active and passive stretches are useful but should be carried out only once medical approval has been given.

Massage

Gentle massage such as effleurage or manual lymphatic drainage can be helpful to stimulate lymphatic drainage and reduce post-operative swelling when applied superior to the knee itself.

Stretching

Active flexion and extension movements within the patient's pain-free range will not only facilitate the lengthening of soft tissue structures to restore typical range of motion at the knee but will also help reduce swelling.

Active Stretches

The stretch shown in figure 5.36 is a good starting point. This could then be progressed to flexion and extension in a seated position. Alternatively, the patient could sit with the knee in extension, resting the calf and foot on a chair or stool to stretch the posterior capsule of the knee (figure 5.39). This is particularly helpful for patients who have been unable to achieve full knee extension; in this position, gravity helps gently stretch the posterior of the joint.

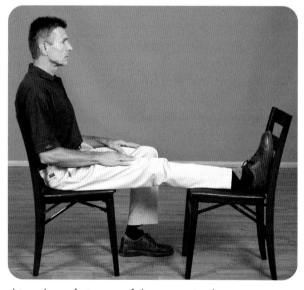

Figure 5.39   Stretching the soft tissues of the posterior knee.

Passive Stretches

A simple passive stretch is performed by facilitating gentle flexion and extension of the knee whilst supporting the lower limb beneath the knee and ankle, as shown in figure 5.40.

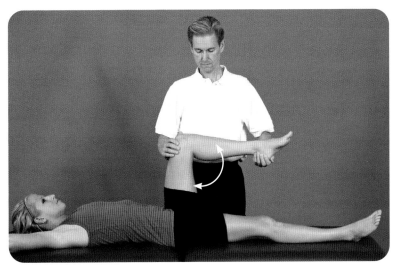

Figure 5.40 Gentle passive flexion of the knee in the supine position.

Passive knee flexion can also be encouraged in the prone position. However, some patients may feel uncomfortable in this position, particularly if they have an anterior scar that they feel anxious about resting on.

Soft Tissue Release

Active assisted STR to the hamstrings is particularly useful as part of the rehabilitation process after surgery to the knee or immobilisation of the knee joint, because it increases knee range of motion and hamstring strength. The hamstrings contract concentrically each time the client actively flexes their knee; they contract eccentrically as the client lowers their knee, thus helping to maintain strength in these muscles.

When the STR technique is used after knee replacement surgery, it may help increase both knee flexion and extension, because the client works within their pain-free range and is likely to increase range at the knee in a way that is safer than post-operative passive stretching.

Strengthening

When someone has been unable to bear weight due to pain prior to surgery, there is likely to be muscle wasting. There is also likely to be atrophy in muscles in cases where surgery required a period of immobilisation or rest. In such cases, strength will be reduced in the entire lower limb, and it will be important to regain this strength. Please see chapter 8 for further information.

Iliotibial Band Friction Syndrome (Runner's Knee)

Iliotibial band friction syndrome is often referred to simply as ITBS or by the lay term *runner's knee*. It is not entirely clear what causes the lateral knee pain experienced by some runners, but some believe the pain is due to the iliotibial band (ITB) of the lateral thigh rubbing against the epicondyle of the femur. Hutchinson and colleagues (2022) provide a clear description of the anatomy and function of the ITB. Kondrup, Gaudreault and Venne (2022) reviewed deep fascia and its role in chronic pain and pathological conditions. They say that ITBS resembles other fascial pathologies and that more research is needed relating to innervation of fascia, inflammation and tissue contracture.

It has been postulated that deep tissue massage, trigger point release and stretching will alleviate the pain of ITBS, and this section provides some ideas for working the lateral side of the thigh. Evidence is limited for stretching of the ITB itself. Because the gluteal muscles insert into the ITB, treatment is likely to be more effective if you treat those muscles also. For more information, please refer to the section on trigger points in the gluteal muscles.

Massage

It is unknown whether massage to the lateral thigh will alleviate runner's knee, especially if the cause is due to biomechanical imbalance. However, it can prove temporarily soothing. Two ways to apply massage to this area involve using your forearm with your client in the three-quarter lying position.

For the first method, begin by standing so you are facing the front of the client. Position your forearm just above the knee; using your other hand for reinforcement, glide slowly and deeply up the lateral thigh, compressing the ITB and vastus lateralis muscle (figure 5.41*a*). An alternative method is to stand behind the client and pull your forearm across the tissues, again from the knee to the thigh (figure 5.41*b*).

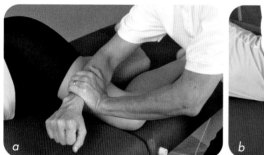 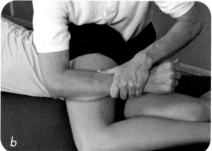

Figure 5.41 Use the forearm to massage the lateral thigh either *(a)* facing your client or *(b)* standing behind them.

TIP

Some clients feel more comfortable with a small, folded towel or cushion beneath their knee on the side you are treating.

Instead of using your forearms on the ITB, a stronger technique is to use reinforced fists. This is a useful technique for working the distal end of the ITB and vastus lateralis. Begin with the client in the three-quarter lying position, and place your fists gently near the knee, avoiding bony structures. Keeping your wrists and elbows as straight as possible, glide firmly towards the hip (figure 5.42).

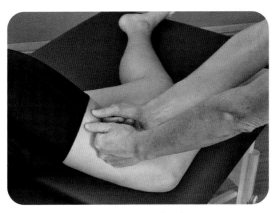

Figure 5.42   Massaging the lateral thigh using the fists.

Trigger Point Release

The ITB is a thickening of the fascia covering the lateral side of the thigh and overlying the vastus lateralis (figure 5.43). Tender spots here are likely to be triggers in this muscle, and they refer pain throughout the side of the thigh from the hip to the knee. Palpate for these triggers with your client in the supine position, turned slightly away from you so that the lateral part of the thigh closest to you is raised off the couch a little. These trigger points are difficult to identify due to the thick fascial covering.

Pavkovich (2015) noted improvements in the Lower Extremity Functional Scale and Quadruple Visual Analogue Scale for four trigger points in the vastus lateralis as well as trigger points in the gluteus maximus, gluteus medius, piriformis and greater trochanter area in a recreational walker with chronic lateral hip and thigh pain. Trigger points were treated with dry needling twice a week for 8 weeks. The patient reported a significant improvement in quality of life in terms of being able to sleep on the affected side, walk farther without pain and stand for extended periods. The author notes that strength in the lower limb improved and postulated that the improvement was a result of the participant having less pain and an improved gait posture.

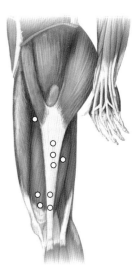

Figure 5.43   Trigger points in the vastus lateralis.

Simple, static pressure to the trigger points can be applied using your fingers, thumbs or an elbow. Some people advocate using a foam roller to deactivate trigger points in the lateral thigh, in which case you would need to instruct your client to rest on a roller (figure 5.44), positioning over sensitive spots on the lateral thigh. However, this can be a difficult position for many people to attain.

As always, it is important to stretch the muscle after trigger point release.

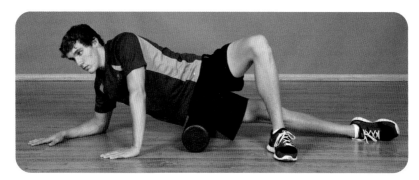

Figure 5.44 Active trigger point release of the lateral thigh using a foam roller.

Stretching

Although a standing stretch performed actively has been popularly advocated by others as a stretch of the ITB and for the treatment of runner's knee, in the author's experience, this is not particularly effective. Clients who wish to help alleviate this condition with the use of stretching are recommended to instead stretch the gluteus maximus and tensor fasciae latae muscles. These muscles insert into the ITB and, when stretched, theoretically reduce tension in the lateral side of the thigh and might therefore reduce the symptoms of runner's knee. Useful passive stretches are included in this section.

Passive Stretches

Myofascial release of the region could be helpful, using the position shown in figure 5.45 with the client in the side-lying position. Be careful when using this stretch, because it requires the client to be positioned close to the edge of the treatment couch.

Passively stretch the gluteal muscles also. If using the supine gluteal stretch shown in figure 5.46, aim to take the knee towards the opposite shoulder, thus stretching the gluteal muscles and lateral thigh simultaneously. In this example, the client's left knee would be moved towards their right shoulder.

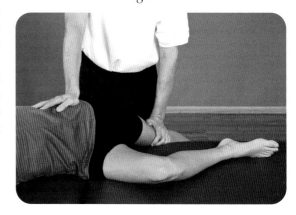

Figure 5.45 Passively tensing the lateral thigh.

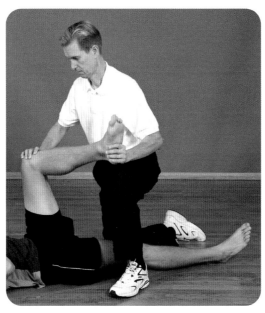

Figure 5.46   Passively stretching the gluteal muscles and lateral thigh.

Soft Tissue Release

Soft tissue release can be a useful way to tense the lateral thigh. With your client in the side-lying position, check that they can flex the knee comfortably; if not, place a small towel or sponge between the client's knee and the edge of the couch. With the knee extended, direct your pressure towards the hip as you gently lock the tissues with soft fists (figure 5.47a). Maintain your lock as your client slowly flexes the knee (figure 5.47b). Select a different lock position that is more proximal than your first and repeat the procedure.

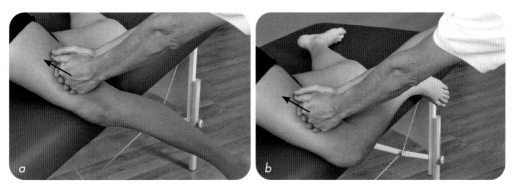

Figure 5.47   (a) Gently lock the iliotibial band with soft fists followed by (b) active knee flexion.

You can modify the active assisted gliding STR used for the calf and tibialis anterior to gliding STR for the lateral thigh. Begin by simply applying a little massage medium, then place your lock just above the knee, gliding from the knee to the hip as your client actively flexes and extends the knee.

Strengthening

Iliotibial band friction syndrome is associated with hip abductor weakness. In a study of 62 people with ITBS, Abdelmowla, Abdelmowla and Fahem (2022) examined the effect of home exercise and function. Half of the participants completed a set of stretches and strengthening exercises once per day, 7 days a week for 8 weeks, performing three sets of 10 repetitions. The objective measurements the researchers used were the Numerical Pain Rating Scale and the Lower Extremity Functional Scale. At 4 weeks and 8 weeks, they found a significant reduction in pain in the exercise group and a significant improvement in function. Please refer to chapter 7 for more information about hip abductor strengthening.

Kinesio Taping

Watcharakhueankhan and colleagues (2022) examined the immediate effects of Kinesio Taping on running biomechanics, muscle activity, and perceived changes in comfort, stability and running performance in healthy runners. Their study found that running mechanics could be altered with the use of Kinesio Taping by reducing activation in the tensor fasciae latae and increasing external rotation of the femur, leading them to conclude that this could be a useful treatment for ITBS.

Placement of a foam roller beneath the lateral thigh and actively rolling along this area has anecdotally been found to be helpful in symptom management.

Genu Recurvatum (Knee Hyperextension)

In the genu recurvatum posture, the degree of knee extension is greater than in the neutral posture. People with this posture sometimes experience patellofemoral pain as the patella is compressed against the underlying tibiofemoral joint, and weight bearing through a hyperextended knee strains the tissues of the posterior knee, leading to an imbalance between the anterior and posterior of the joint and increasing the likelihood of injury.

Education

One of the most helpful things you can do is to educate your client about this posture. Instruct your client about maintaining good postural alignment, helping them to identify those times when they stand with the knees locked out in the hyperextended posture. A person with hyperextended knees needs to be conscious of knee postures during everyday activities. They need to practise good knee alignment in static postures, taking particular care with standing postures by avoiding locking out the knee. They also need to avoid placing the ankles on a footstool when seated, because this allows the knees to sag into extension, stretching posterior tissues. They should also practise good knee alignment during dynamic functions such as standing up from a sitting position and when stair climbing.

When working with a client who engages in regular stretching, advise them to avoid exercises and stretches that force the knee into extension. For example, they should take care with standing hamstring and calf stretches.

Taping

Rather than preventing hyperextension, the purpose of taping is to provide sensory feedback to help your client identify when they have a tendency to hyperextend. This may be particularly useful when treating dancers with hypermobility syndrome (Knight 2011). Ultimately, self-correction of the posture is preferable to reliance on tape, which should be used only in the short term whilst your client is learning to avoid hyperextension. Tape can be applied in a variety of ways, such as a single wide strip (figure 5.48a), two narrower strips (figure 5.48b) or a cross (figure 5.48c). Whichever method you choose, apply the tape with the knee in a neutral position. Rather than attempting this with your client standing, ask them to lie face down, where the knee usually rests in a neutral position.

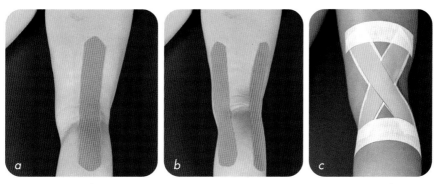

Figure 5.48 Taping for genu recurvatum using (a) one or (b) two pieces of tape or (c) applying tape in a cross shape.

Massage

In the genu recurvatum posture, the quadriceps are shortened with respect to the hamstrings, pressing the patella against the underlying bony tibiofemoral joint. Massage can be used to help relax and lengthen the quadriceps – for example, by using a gliding stroke from just superior to the patella to the proximal end of the thigh using your forearm (figure 5.49a) or gripping and squeezing the muscle (figure 5.49b).

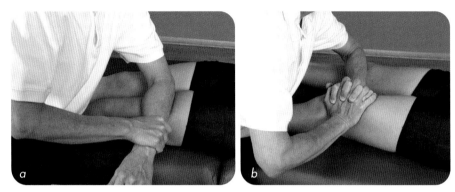

Figure 5.49 Apply deep tissue massage to the quadriceps by (a) gliding with the forearm or (b) gripping.

Stretching

In this posture, the quadriceps are shortened relative to the hamstrings. Therefore, stretching of this muscle group can help reduce the imbalance between the anterior and posterior muscles.

Passive Stretches

Examples of passive stretches are shown in figures 5.50a and 5.50b.

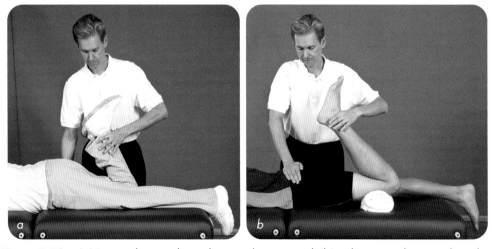

Figure 5.50 (a) Passively stretching the quadriceps and (b) enhancing the stretch with use of a towel.

Active Stretches

Figures 5.51a and 5.51b are examples of useful active stretches. When your client is in the standing position, remember to instruct them to avoid locking and hyperextending the leg they are standing on. One way to avoid hyperextension of the supporting leg is to stand with that knee slightly flexed.

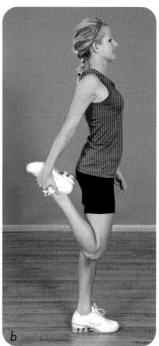

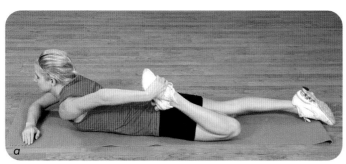

Figure 5.51 An active quadriceps stretch in the *(a)* prone and *(b)* standing positions.

Strengthening

If you think it falls within your professional remit, provide exercises to strengthen the knee flexors. These could include regular hamstring and calf strengthening or asking your client to perform slight knee flexion against the gentle resistance of your hands placed just beneath the knee (figure 5.52) within a small range of motion. Take care of your own posture when facilitating this exercise, perhaps by asking your client to stand on a raised platform so that you do not have to stoop too much.

Chapter 8 provides additional exercises on knee strengthening, and chapter 9 provides exercises on balance, all of which can be useful for clients needing to manage knee hyperextension.

Referral to a Specialist

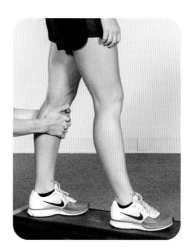

Figure 5.52 Handhold for facilitating knee strengthening in a specific range of motion.

Consider referring your client to a podiatrist, who may have suggestions for treatment to limit the extent of hyperextension during daily activities. For example, using a slightly elevated heel creates knee flexion during walking, which slows the gait but can be helpful in preventing hyperextension. Use of orthotics under the medial border of the foot can help limit subtalar pronation, a posture associated with genu recurvatum. Ankle Foot Orthoses

(AFO), rigid ankle and foot boots, are sometimes prescribed to help correct genu recurvatum whilst walking; however, although these reduce the energy requirement of walking, they do not always reduce extensor movement at the knee (Kerrigan, Deming, and Holden 1996).

Finally, if your client is engaged in sporting activity, you could also consider referral to a sports therapist for sport-specific drills. These kinds of drills can help your client master a flexed knee position during fast, dynamic movements and therefore reduce the likelihood of injury. Your client should consider protecting the knees against hyperextension during sporting activities, especially those involving impact, such as jumping.

Discuss which forms of sporting activity may be most suitable to someone with genu recurvatum posture. Prevention of knee hyperextension requires focused control of the joint and could be aggravated by sports involving fast movements. This posture may be disadvantageous to participation in field sports such as rugby, football, hockey and lacrosse (Bloomfield, Ackland, and Elliott 1994). It is likely to be disadvantageous for participation in jumping sports and sports that involve excessive loading of the lower limb. Clients with hyperextended knees would be better suited to activities such as tai chi, where movements are slow and controlled, rather than high-impact sports involving frequent changes of direction, such as racquet sports. Simple balancing exercises are beneficial to these clients because they adopt a neutral knee position and attempt to maintain it.

Genu Flexum (Flexed Knee)

A person may have a genu flexum knee posture for a variety of reasons. It may occur simply through the retention of a flexed knee position for long periods of time, as in people who are sedentary. It may also occur after surgery when posterior knee structures tighten, combined with prolonged bed rest and lack of movement of the knee. As with hyperextension of the knee, you can help by educating your client with regards to how to treat this posture. For example, advise them to avoid sitting for prolonged periods with the knees flexed. If they have a seated job, advise them to take short breaks and stand every hour to stretch the back of the legs. In some cases, it might be useful for a client to temporarily avoid sports that might perpetuate a flexed knee posture, such as rowing and cycling.

Caution is needed when attempting to address genu flexum after knee surgery and when working with clients who use wheelchairs or spend much of their time in a chair, such as someone who might be frail or recovering from illness or injury.

For each of the techniques suggested, consider whether deep pressure (as might be used when applying STR or addressing trigger points) is contraindicated for your client. Recognise that intervention may be limited for clients in whom genu flexum results from abnormal high tone (e.g., spasticity associated with cerebral palsy).

Myofascial Release

Passively release posterior knee tissues using the myofascial release technique. This is an ideal technique to use for this posture, in which tissues on the back of the knee are tensed and pressure into the back of the knee must be avoided because of the presence of the popliteal artery and lymph nodes. A simple cross-hand technique could work well here, with one hand placed superior to the knee and one inferior to it.

Massage

Massage can be used to encourage relaxation and lengthening of the hamstrings (figure 5.53) and gastrocnemius (figure 5.54), the two muscles that cross the posterior knee joint along with the popliteus. Remember to avoid direct pressure to the knee joint itself. Treat any trigger points that you find in posterior tissues using localised static pressure and taking care not to press directly into the popliteal space.

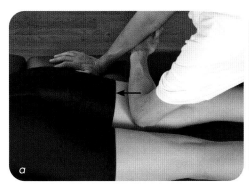 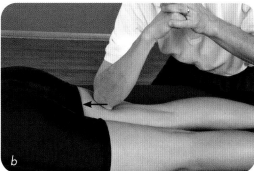

Figure 5.53 *(a)* Massage to the hamstrings using the forearm, with *(b)* use of the elbow to deactivate trigger points.

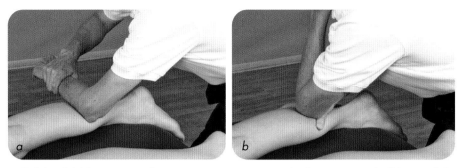

Figure 5.54 *(a)* Massage to the gastrocnemius using the forearm, with *(b)* use of the elbow to deactivate trigger points.

Soft Tissue Release

Soft tissue release is useful for a client with flexed knees because it permits you or your client to work within a range of knee flexion postures, stretching localised tissues only as far as is comfortable. Active STR to the hamstrings (figures 5.55a and 5.55b) is preferable, because once the client has pressed the tennis ball against their thigh, contraction of the opposing muscle group (in this case, the quadriceps) helps reduce tone in the hamstrings. For clients who find it difficult to rest supine, STR can be performed seated (figure 5.56). However, this requires the knee to be extended against gravity, and this is more difficult than knee extension in the supine position.

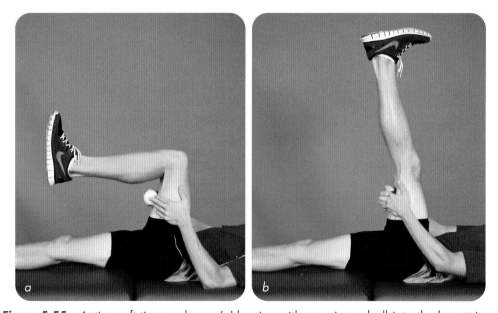

Figure 5.55 Active soft tissue release *(a)* begins with pressing a ball into the hamstrings and *(b)* helps reduce tone in the hamstrings, and therefore knee flexion, through contraction of the quadriceps.

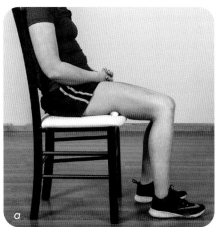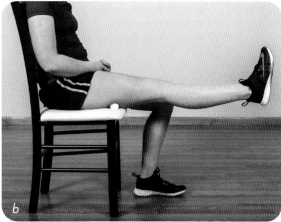

Figure 5.56 Active soft tissue release in the seated position begins with *(a)* compression of the hamstrings using a ball, followed by *(b)* knee extension.

Stretching

The hamstrings and soleus are shortened in the genu flexum posture. Stretching these (and also strengthening the quadriceps) may help reduce the effects of this posture on the joint.

Passive Stretches

There are many ways to do this, including simple stretches held at the end of the existing range (figure 5.57). One advantage of a simple supine hamstring stretch is that it can be performed with the knee flexed. Instead of passively flexing the hip at the end of the range, ask your client to extend the knee. Contraction of the quadriceps will facilitate relaxation of the hamstrings, increasing knee extension without the need for further hip flexion.

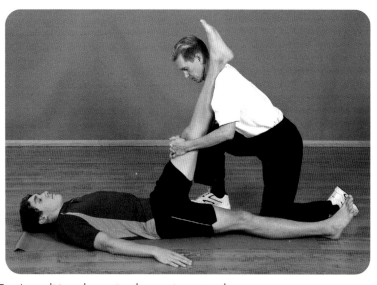

Figure 5.57 A traditional passive hamstring stretch.

Your client can help by resting in positions likely to stretch the posterior knee tissues. For example, when using a footrest, the posterior knee is stretched through gravity (figure 5.58). Notice the tension in the tissues of the person's right thigh in the figure.

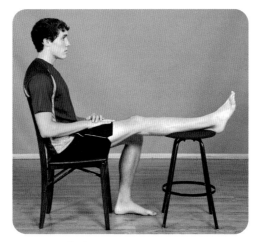

Figure 5.58　Letting gravity stretch the posterior tissues in a sitting position.

Active Stretches

Active stretching of the hamstrings (figure 5.59) and gastrocnemius (figure 5.60) is useful. Using a towel (figure 5.61) helps stretch both the hamstrings and gastrocnemius together.

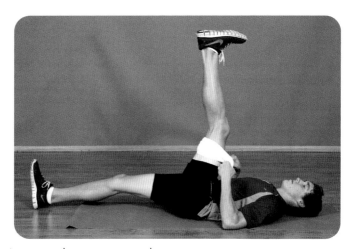

Figure 5.59　An active hamstring stretch.

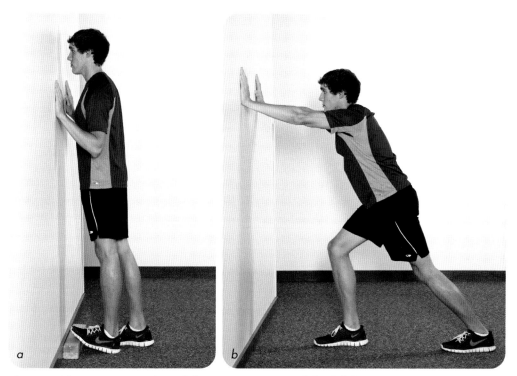

Figure 5.60   Active stretches of the gastrocnemius of the left leg.

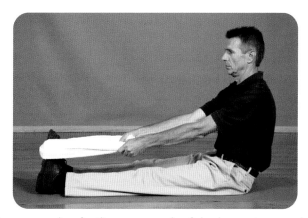

Figure 5.61   Using a towel to facilitate a stretch of the hamstrings and gastrocnemius at the same time.

Another technique is for the client to rest in the prone position, with their feet off the couch; a light weight can be added to the ankle. This too will stretch posterior tissues of the knee, but take care when using the prone position so as not to injure the front of the knee against the side of the couch or bed. The prone position is not suitable for clients with patellofemoral conditions in which compression of the patella could be aggravating.

Genu Varum (Bow-Leggedness)

It is important to recognise that where a change to bone tissue has occurred, such as bowing of the femur or tibia or both, non-surgical intervention is limited. Where bow-leggedness appears to be postural only, with little or no anatomical change, it is helpful to encourage your client to identify and avoid movements that may aggravate this posture (e.g., shifting weight to the affected leg and permitting the knee to bow outwards). If possible, the client should avoid sports that involve high impact or excessive loading, because these increase stress through the knee joint, further compressing and tensing structures. They might consider wearing a knee brace when taking part in sporting activities. This may alleviate pain during weight bearing and may lessen the chances of injury.

Taping

Although controversial, anecdotal evidence suggests that taping may be helpful in training gluteal muscles. The method shown in figure 5.62 is based on that recommended by Langendoen and Sertel (2011). One at a time, apply two strips of tape from the proximal anterior thigh, running them posteriorly to mimic the direction of gluteal fibres.

Taping the lateral side of the knee joint (figure 5.63) is a temporary measure usually used to address knee pain. It can be useful in providing sensory feedback to clients but will have little if any impact on anatomical (rather than postural) genu varum. One approach is to tape as if for a lateral collateral ligament sprain, where your aim is to prevent further gapping of the lateral side of the knee. In this case, you would attach a horizontal fixing strip above and below the knee and then make a cross shape between them, using two further pieces of tape, aiming for the centre of the cross to fall over the lateral collateral ligament. Some therapists tape with the client standing, but it can be helpful for the client to be in a side-lying position with the affected knee uppermost. In this way, gravity helps reduce the gapping on the lateral side of the knee before taping.

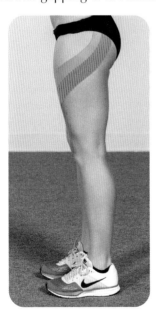

Figure 5.62 Taping the gluteal muscles to facilitate external rotation of the hip.

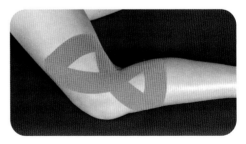

Figure 5.63 Taping the lateral aspect of the knee.

Massage

Massaging muscles that are relatively short could be beneficial, but similar to stretching, it may have a limited effect with regards to the genu varum posture. Note that massaging the adductors with your client in the supine position can cause discomfort, which sometimes tenses the lateral side of the knee, so a side-lying position can be preferable (figure 5.64).

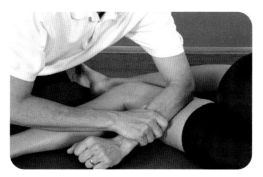

Figure 5.64   Massage to the adductors with the client in a side-lying position.

Trigger Point Release

It can be helpful to release trigger points in the tensor fasciae latae (figure 5.65a) and the anterior fibres of the gluteus medius (figure 5.65b). You will need to experiment with the best position to access these muscles. For example, the gluteus medius might also be accessed posteriorly (figure 5.65c).

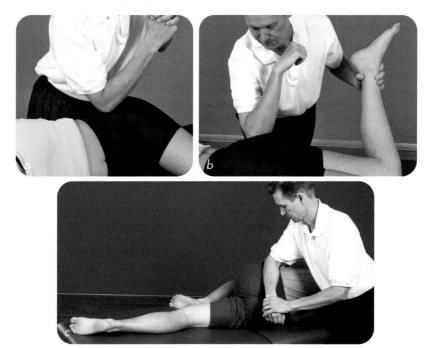

Figure 5.65   Releasing trigger points in (a) the tensor fasciae latae and gluteus medius in the (b) prone and (c) side-lying positions.

Stretching

Although it may have a limited effect, stretching muscles that are relatively short in the genu varum posture (the internal rotators of the hip, the quadriceps and the gracilis) could be beneficial.

Passive Stretches

Figure 5.66 shows three ways to stretch the internal rotators of the hip passively. One of the challenges in doing this is that the supine stretches (figure 5.66a and 5.66b) usually advocated for these muscles promote gapping of the lateral side of the knee, so they need to be performed with care.

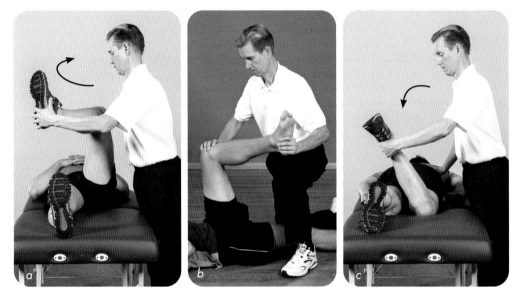

Figure 5.66 Passively stretching the internal rotators of the hip in the (a, b) supine and (c) prone positions.

When passively stretching the gracilis, take care not to strain the outside of the knee, because this has a tendency to become compressed as the hip is abducted. Experiment with different positions (figure 5.67)

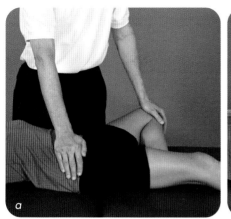
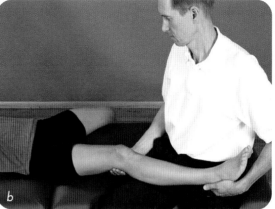

Figure 5.67 Positions for passively stretching the gracilis: *(a)* with the knee flexed and the opposite side of the pelvis fixed and *(b)* with the knee extended and one leg hooked over the table to add stability.

Active Stretches

Figure 5.68 shows two ways to stretch the internal rotators of the hip actively.

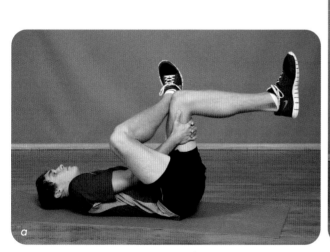
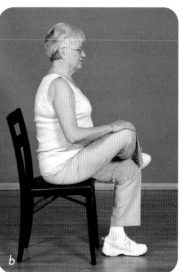

Figure 5.68 Active stretching of the internal rotators of the hip in the *(a)* supine and *(b)* seated positions.

Strengthening

To correct postural bow legs, Kendall, McCreary and Provance (1993) advocate standing with the feet about 5 centimetres (2 in.) apart and the knees comfortably relaxed, then tightening the buttock muscles to experience a lifting of the arches of the feet. Transfer a slight amount of weight onto the lateral sides of the feet, then tighten the buttocks further in an attempt to rotate the legs slightly outward and have the patellae facing forwards. Strengthening of the external hip rotators using exercises such as prone hip extension and bridging is helpful, as might be strengthening of the tibialis posterior and the long toe flexor muscles. Please see chapter 7 for more information on hip strengthening and chapter 9 for toe flexor strengthening. Shams Abrigh and Moghaddami (2020) reported success with use of a strengthening programme when used with teenage footballers with genu varum knee posture. To determine the effectiveness of the programme, the authors measured the distance between the condyles of the participants' knees. They used small sets of high-repetition exercises for 8 weeks. In the exercise group, they reported a significant difference in pretest and posttest genu varum measurements. However, the effect of strengthening on knee posture is likely to be minimal in the adult population when joint posture is more fixed, and the high numbers of repetitions required for the exercises is likely to affect adherence to such a programme.

Podiatry

Consider referring your client to a podiatrist, who may be able to offer specialist advice. For example, angled insoles can be used to transfer the load from the medial to the lateral compartment of the knee and perhaps alter the tibiofemoral angle. Lateral forefoot and rearfoot wedge insoles have been used to facilitate foot pronation (Gross 1995).

Genu Valgum (Knock Knees)

You learned in chapter 1 that in the genu valgum posture, the tensor fasciae latae and the ITB are compressed along with tissues of the lateral leg compartment. Because there is often structural change in the knee joint, it is important to educate your client as to the limitations of soft tissue techniques with regards to changing this posture. There are, however, useful tips you can provide to help reduce pain.

Education

As with the genu varum knee posture, it is important to educate your client with regards to how they might avoid stressing the structures of their knee. For example, they need to identify and avoid lazy standing postures that aggravate the genu valgum stance. This sometimes occurs when tired or in the habit of shifting weight onto one leg. They should avoid resting the feet around chair legs when sitting (figure 5.69), because this strains the medial side of the knee and ankle. If possible, they should avoid sports that involve high impact, because these increase stress through the knee joint, further compressing and tensing the structures. A knee brace is an option. Note that this may alleviate pain during weight bearing but will not redress bony structures.

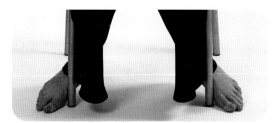

Figure 5.69   Avoid hooking the feet around chair legs when sitting.

Taping

You can tape the medial side of the knee joint, but note that this is a temporary measure usually used for overcoming pain and will not provide long-term correction of a genu valgum knee. One way to apply tape is as if you were taping a medial collateral sprain, attempting to orientate the centre of a cross over the medial collateral ligament (figure 5.70).

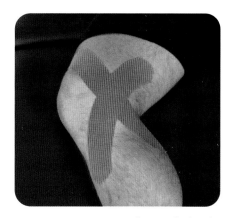

Figure 5.70   Taping the medial side of the knee.

167

TIP

A tip here is to position your client in a side-lying position, resting on the affected limb. In this position, the medial collateral ligament will be uppermost, but the knee will be supported by the couch. You can apply gentle pressure as you apply the tape, taking the knee into a more neutral position if this is comfortable for the client.

Massage

Massage the gracilis if this is found to be shortened. If you choose to treat your client in the side-lying position with the client resting on the affected limb, the adductors will be accessible, yet the knee will be supported by the couch (figure 5.71), and you can massage the gracilis without the risk of gapping the knee joint further.

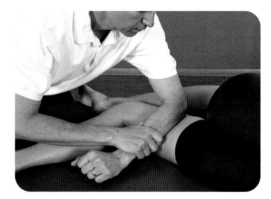

Figure 5.71 Massage to the adductors in the side-lying position.

Trigger Point Release

Static pressure to the tensor fasciae latae (figure 5.72) can be used to address any trigger points found in this muscle (figure 5.73) and to encourage relaxation and lengthening of the tissue. Using a tennis ball to trigger and stretch the tensor fasciae latae can be useful, but in practice, it can be a difficult position for many clients to achieve without compromising the knee joint in the process (figure 5.74). One solution is to tape the knee joint before the client attempts to use the ball or for the client to wear a knee brace whilst using the ball.

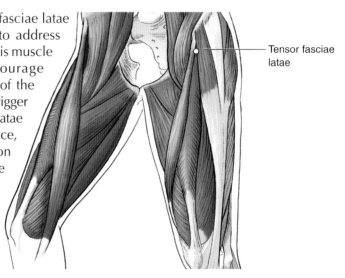

Tensor fasciae latae

Figure 5.72 Tensor fasciae latae trigger point.

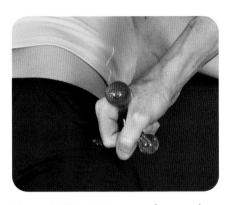

Figure 5.73 Using a tool to apply static pressure to the tensor fasciae latae.

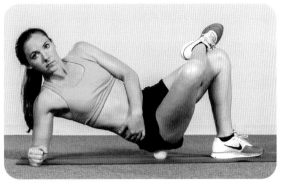

Figure 5.74 The position needed to self-trigger the tensor fasciae latae using a tennis ball can be challenging.

Myofascial Release and Soft Tissue Release

In the genu varum posture, the ITB is shortened relative to a neutral posture, and the vastus lateralis can develop trigger points (figure 5.75). Figure 5.76 shows a useful position to apply myofascial release to the ITB, and STR is also useful in releasing tension in this tissue.

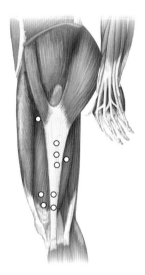

Figure 5.75 Trigger points in the vastus lateralis.

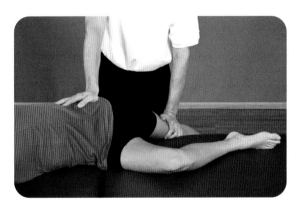

Figure 5.76 A useful position to apply myofascial release to the lateral thigh.

To apply STR, work with your client in the side-lying position. Gently lock the tissues with the client's knee in extension (figure 5.77a), and then ask the client to flex their knee (figure 5.77b).

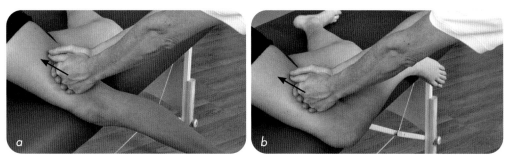

Figure 5.77 Applying soft tissue release to the lateral thigh begins *(a)* with the knee in extension followed by *(b)* active knee flexion.

In the genu valgum posture, the knees fall inwards and the ankle everts. A consequence of this is that the peroneal (fibular) muscles are in a shortened rather than neutral position and can develop trigger points (figure 5.78). Because the degree of ankle inversion and eversion is less than that of plantar flexion and extension, STR can be used to release trigger points in the peroneal muscles (figure 5.79). With your client in the side-lying position and the ankle everted, lock the tissues at the proximal end of the muscle (figure 5.79a). Maintaining your lock, ask your client to invert their ankle (figure 5.79b).

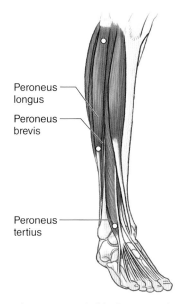

Peroneus longus

Peroneus brevis

Peroneus tertius

Figure 5.78 Trigger points in the peroneal (fibular) muscles.

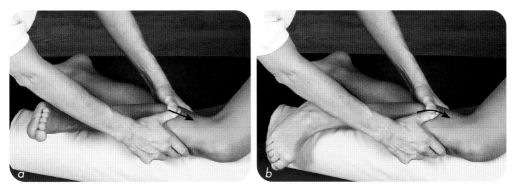

Figure 5.79 Soft tissue release to the peroneal muscles begins with *(a)* a lock applied to the proximal end of the tissues whilst the client has their ankle in eversion, followed by *(b)* active inversion of the ankle as the therapist maintains the lock.

Stretching

Stretching of the lateral thigh is challenging. Because the gluteal muscles insert into the ITB, it may be more effective to stretch them, either passively (figure 5.80*a*) or actively (figure 5.80*b*).

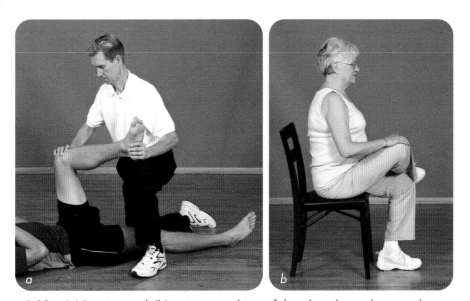

Figure 5.80 *(a)* Passive and *(b)* active stretching of the gluteal muscles to reduce tension in the iliotibial band.

Podiatry

Consider referring your client to a podiatrist, who may be able to offer specialist advice. For example, angled insoles can be used to transfer the load from the lateral to the medial compartment of the knee and perhaps alter the tibiofemoral angle. Use of medial wedge insoles has been found to reduce pain and improve function in patients with valgus knee osteoarthritis (Rodrigues et al. 2008).

Quick Questions

1. Which muscle can someone actively contract to help reduce the sensation of cramping in the calf?

2. What is a more accurate term for *shin splints*?

3. When preparing to work on trigger points to the peroneal (fibular) muscles, of which nerve should you be careful in the region of the head of the fibula?

4. When working with someone with osteoarthritis in the knee, why should soft tissue techniques only be used in conjunction with therapeutic exercise?

5. In which knee posture is tape applied for the treatment of genu recurvatum – knee flexion, knee extension or a neutral knee posture?

6

Foot and Ankle

Learning Outcomes

After reading this chapter, you should be able to do the following:

- Teach a client simple range-of-motion exercises after an ankle sprain and as part of ankle fracture rehabilitation.
- Describe which techniques are appropriate for the treatment of Achilles tendinopathy.
- Explain why the use of active dorsiflexion may be more effective than passive dorsiflexion.
- Describe which stretches are appropriate for the treatment of plantar fasciitis.
- Demonstrate soft tissue release to the fibular muscles.
- List the foot and ankle conditions for which strengthening exercises are useful.

In this chapter, you will learn which hands-on techniques are appropriate for two acute injuries: a lateral ankle sprain (the most common injury affecting the ankle) and an ankle fracture. By contrast, you will also discover how to treat Achilles tendinopathy. Unlike a sprain or a fracture, an Achilles tendinopathy is not usually an immediate injury but a condition that develops over time. After a sprain or a fracture, the ankle and foot can become stiff, depending on what treatment has been undertaken; therefore, this chapter has a section on how to treat a stiff ankle, and stiffness in the feet is covered in a section on plantar fasciitis, another common condition that is problematic for many people. This chapter also discusses four common foot postures: pes planus, pes cavus, pes valgus and pes varus. Although hands-on techniques cannot significantly alter the posture of the foot, they can be used to alleviate resulting muscle pain, so the chapter has sections on all four postures. For all conditions, strengthening is important; please refer to chapter 9 for ankle and foot strengthening exercises.

Ankle Sprains

An ankle sprain is the wrenching and tearing of ligaments on either the lateral or medial side of the ankle joint, sometimes with damage to the anterior of the joint capsule. The most common form of sprain is an inversion sprain, in which the lateral ligaments are damaged. Less common is an eversion sprain, in which the strong deltoid ligament on the medial side of the ankle is torn. There is pain, swelling and in some cases, bruising, usually resulting in the person having to limp due to an inability to bear weight through the ankle joint. In serious inversion sprains, there may be an avulsion fracture to the fifth metatarsal as the fibularis brevis muscle is wrenched from its insertion. With severe eversion sprains, damage to the distal end of the fibula sometimes occurs when sharp eversion of the foot crushes or snaps that end of the bone.

A Dutch consensus statement (Vuurberg et al. 2018) developed by a multidisciplinary research panel recommends that rest, ice, compression and elevation (RICE), along with immobilisation, should not be used in the treatment of ankle sprains, that supervised exercise programmes are preferable to passive modalities and that exercise should begin as soon as possible. However, the National Institute for Health and Clinical Excellence (2020) continues to recommend the RICE protocol, with the addition of 'P' – protect from further injury (PRICE) – as a self-management approach within the first 24 to 48 hours after injury. Therefore, it is important that you use hands-on techniques only as an adjunct to exercises and not as a stand-alone treatment.

With regards to hands-on techniques, massage and passive stretching are best avoided in the acute and sub-acute stages of the sprain, because it is important to gain a balance between keeping the ankle mobile and avoiding retearing soft tissues that are repairing. However, movement of the ankle is important, because this helps the collagen that is being laid down to realign in a more optimal pattern than if the ankle is completely immobilised.

Education

Wikstrom and colleagues (2021) conducted a systematic review of lateral ankle sprains and risk of reinjury. Their review included 19 studies with a total of 6,567 patients and concluded that there is strong evidence that having had a previous lateral ankle sprain is a risk factor for subsequent re-sprain. Interestingly, they reported that there are barriers to rehabilitation, one of which is the erroneous public perception that ankle sprains are inconsequential injuries that do not require rehabilitation. Part of your approach when dealing with clients with an ankle sprain is to provide education in this regard.

Active Ankle Movement

With caution, it is important to begin a gentle ankle movement programme sooner rather than later, because this may help realign collagen fibres in such a way that fibrous adhesions are less likely to occur. Weight bearing should be avoided initially, and movement should be well within a client's pain-free range. Figure 6.1 shows the position most beneficial for the rehabilitation of ankle sprains and in which active movements should be performed.

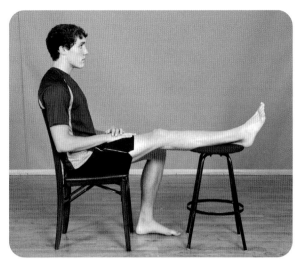

Figure 6.1 Resting position in which to perform active movements of the ankle.

The aim of your initial treatment might be to help the client maintain (and later improve) range of motion in the ankle. It is important that all ranges of movement are restored. Figure 6.2 shows two of these movements: dorsiflexion (a) and plantar flexion (c), compared to a neutral position (b). Figure 6.3 shows the other two ankle movements, inversion and eversion. Instruct your client in performing gentle dorsiflexion and plantar flexion with the foot elevated as shown in figure 6.1, stressing that this should be done within a pain-free range. Later, introduce the movements of eversion and inversion. Dorsiflexion and plantar flexion are used first, because the ankle naturally falls into plantar flexion at rest; if the foot is allowed to remain in this position, it will lead to stiffening of the posterior ankle joint and shortening of muscles in the posterior compartment of the leg. Dorsiflexion and plantar flexion are also the easiest ankle movements. Movements of eversion and inversion are harder for most clients to perform, yet they are important to include at some stage of the rehabilitative process, because they will help restore range of motion in the joint.

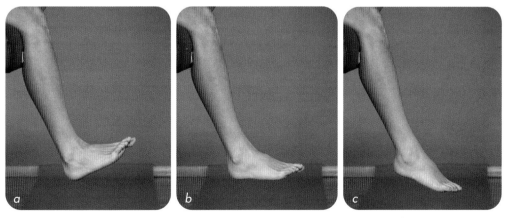

Figure 6.2 The ankle joint (a) dorsiflexed, (b) neutral and (c) plantar flexed.

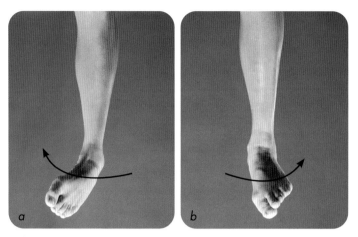

Figure 6.3 Ankle *(a)* inversion and *(b)* eversion.

> **TIP**
>
> Lying supine is an excellent position in which to perform the ankle range-of-motion exercises, because it facilitates lymphatic drainage and thus helps reduce swelling.

Massage

Only extremely light massage in the form of effleurage is advised in the early stages of an ankle sprain. Your client may be hypersensitive to touch in the early stages of repair, but once they can tolerate gentle active movement of the ankle, you could apply extremely light effleurage in the prone position with the knee flexed. In this position, gravity and effleurage from ankle to knee will help reduce swelling of the ankle.

If the ankle has been immobilised after a sprain, with no active range-of-motion exercises, the client may experience a stiffening of the joint as soft tissues shorten and adhere to one another. In this case, you could follow the rehabilitation process described in the section on stiff ankles.

Strengthening

Please see chapter 9 for details of appropriate balance and ankle strengthening exercises.

Braces

In a systematic review of evidence-based treatment choices for acute lateral ankle sprains, Altomare and colleagues (2022) found some evidence to support the use of braces, with a preference for flexible ankle braces because these allowed an earlier return to daily activities.

Ankle Fracture

An ankle fracture is an acute injury accompanied by immediate pain and swelling. Fractures can occur spontaneously in people with osteoporosis. The distal ends of the tibia and fibula or the talus bone of the ankle may be broken. There is usually damage to ligaments of the joint, resulting in swelling of the foot and ankle and sometimes the leg also. Massage and stretching are contraindicated in the acute stage of an ankle fracture. In the sub-acute stage, pain and swelling are reduced, but the ankle is far from being healed, so caution is required.

Active Ankle Movement

Gentle, active movements to maintain and improve range of motion may be helpful, provided there are no complications and you have medical approval. It is not always possible to perform active range of motion treatments if the ankle is immobilised (e.g., in a cast or brace). However, if movements are possible, treat the ankle as you would for a sub-acute ankle sprain. Advise the client to perform active range-of-motion stretches (see figures 6.2 and 6.3) and to avoid weight-bearing stretches.

TIP

Even when patients have been given medical approval to carry out gentle movements of the ankle, they are often fearful of doing so, perhaps believing it will result in reinjury. You can reassure your client that discomfort is likely as a normal part of the healing process but that extreme pain is not. Progress is usually made when you encourage your clients to begin with slow and gentle movements.

Stretching

Remember that immobilisation of the ankle will result in decreased mobility in joints of the foot and toes. Thus, once the fracture is healed, it is important to mobilise and stretch these joints, using stretches suggested in the section on plantar fasciitis and stiff feet later in this chapter.

Strengthening

Loss of lower limb strength is common after an ankle fracture. Therefore, exercises to regain strength and balance are essential. Please see chapter 9 for details on these exercises.

Active Controlled Motion

The term *active controlled motion* (ACM) is somewhat misleading, because it refers to use of a device to perform continuous passive movement. In a randomised controlled trial, Jansen and colleagues (2018) investigated the use of ACM in early rehabilitation and found that it improved outcomes after ankle fractures. Their study involved 50 patients with unstable ankle fractures and the need for only partial weight bearing for 6 weeks. They compared physiotherapy alone with physiotherapy combined with ACM and found that the group receiving ACM had better outcomes across all the questionnaires that were used, better balance and an earlier return to work than the group that received only physiotherapy.

Achilles Tendinopathy

The Achilles tendon is the largest tendon in the body, and the strongest. Blood supply to the tendon is poor. Achilles tendinopathy is usually due to overuse of and excessive stress on the tendon and involves changes in the tendon. Overloading can lead to inflammation and tendon degeneration. This condition is not restricted to people engaged in sporting activity; overload can occur for other reasons, such as one's occupation. Overpronation of the foot has been suggested as a contributing factor. There is usually pain in the tendon on weight bearing after awakening, and in some cases, there may be swelling. The injury is often aggravated by repetitive movement and may therefore limit your client from exercising.

A stiff Achilles tendon that lacks pliability may increase a person's risk of tendinopathy. Therefore, any techniques aimed at reducing tension in the tendon and increasing pliability are beneficial: massage, trigger point release, soft tissue release and both active and passive stretching. Additionally, the fascia of the tendon and calf is concurrent with that of the posterior thigh and foot. Therefore, massage, stretching and trigger point release to the hamstrings and foot are also very helpful. Please see the sections on tight hamstrings (in chapter 4) and plantar fasciitis (later in this chapter) for these techniques.

Education

Before you begin any hands-on treatment, it is important to help your client to identify and reduce activities that are causing overload to the tendon. You will likely need to educate your client with regards to how they might modify their physical activity.

Massage

Massage to the calf is helpful prior to stretching, because this helps reduce tension and improve pliability in the soft tissues into which the Achilles tendon inserts. Apply any of the techniques described in the section on the treatment of tight calf muscles in chapter 5. Also helpful is massage to the hamstrings (chapter 4) and the plantar aspect of the foot (as described in the section on plantar fasciitis in this chapter). There is limited evidence for the use of friction, but anecdotally, this has been reported as useful when the condition has become chronic.

Trigger Point Release

Release of tension in the calf may help with the management of Achilles tendinopathy. The trigger point release techniques described in the section on the treatment of tight calf muscles in chapter 5 are appropriate. Also helpful are deactivation of the trigger points to the hamstrings (chapter 4) and those used in plantar fasciitis (later in this chapter).

Stretching

Both active and passive stretches are contraindicated in the acute stage of Achilles tendinopathy. In the sub-acute stage, both pain and inflammation (if there is any) may have subsided, yet the condition persists. Passive and active stretches are both helpful in the treatment of this condition. It is important to perform passive stretches to both the gastrocnemius and the soleus muscles. Any of the techniques described in the section on the treatment of tight calf muscles in chapter 5 are appropriate. Stretches described in the section on the treatment of tight hamstrings (chapter 4) and plantar fasciitis (later in this chapter) are useful additions.

Soft Tissue Release

In sub-acute stages of Achilles tendinopathy, soft tissue release (STR) may be helpful. The method of applying STR to the calf described in the section on the treatment of tight calf muscles in chapter 5 is useful. Soft tissue release for tight hamstrings (chapter 4) is also helpful.

Strengthening

Unlike the treatment of an ankle sprain, for which weight bearing is to be avoided initially, weight bearing may be safe for sub-acute and chronic tendinopathy and is possibly advantageous, because the Achilles tendon can withstand remarkably high forces. Strengthening in the form of controlled tendon loading is particularly important. Chapter 9 also describes important exercises designed to strengthen this tendon.

Referral to a Specialist

Because overpronation of the foot has been linked to Achilles tendinopathy, please see the section on pes valgus in this chapter for treatment ideas. Referral to a specialist (e.g., a physical therapist, osteopath or chiropractor) for gait analysis may be helpful. If the condition is the result of joint dysfunction, referral to a specialist for joint mobilisation may also be of benefit.

Stiff Ankle

Many people suffer from stiff ankles. This condition may result from a sedentary lifestyle or direct immobilisation of the lower limb due to serious injury or surgery. Clients sometimes complain of stiffness resulting from a previous injury for which there was little or no intervention; function has been restored, but limitations in range of motion remain. Any modality that improves pliability of soft tissues and movement of the ankle joint is likely to be helpful.

Massage

General massage to the whole leg and the ankle is helpful to mobilise tissues before stretching.

Stretching

Both active and passive stretches are helpful to increase range of motion in the ankle and reduce the sensation of stiffness. It is important to first determine whether there is a reduction in any particular range of motion or whether the entire ankle is stiff. Simply pointing the toes may increase plantar flexion (figure 6.4a), but if active flexion is limited, passive stretching may be required (figure 6.4b). Remember that the ankle naturally falls into plantar flexion at rest, and it is important not to passively overstretch the soft tissues of the anterior aspect of this joint when using this position.

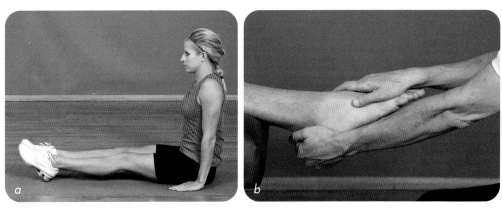

Figure 6.4 *(a)* Active and *(b)* passive stretches to increase plantar flexion.

Eversion may be particularly challenging to achieve. Placing a towel beneath the lateral side of the foot (figure 6.5a) and simply standing in this position helps increase the movement of eversion by stretching the invertor muscles. Passive stretches are useful if a client has not been bearing weight for a while and may have lost their sense of balance (figure 6.5b).

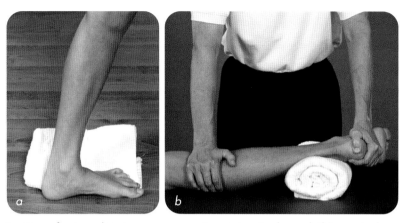

Figure 6.5   Use of a towel to increase eversion *(a)* actively and *(b)* passively.

TIP
_____

Passive stretching to increase eversion is best performed with the client in a side-lying position (figure 6.5*b*). Use a small towel, rolled or folded to form a pad to elevate the ankle.

_____

The preinjury range of dorsiflexion is relatively easy to regain, because the ankle is
at a 90-degree angle to the floor when we stand. Therefore, reducing plantar flexion to
achieve a 90-degree angle at the ankle joint simply requires the client to stand. If your
client is bedbound but intends to walk in the future, passive stretching of the ankle into
dorsiflexion will be helpful. The active and passive stretches shown in the section on
treating tight calf muscles in chapter 5 are all useful.

A common mistake made when trying to regain dorsiflexion to overcome a stiff ankle
is to limit the range of motion to 90 degrees. Although this facilitates standing with
the sole of the foot flat on the floor, it limits normal walking. Increasing the range of
dorsiflexion from 90 degrees is important. When we rest, the ankle naturally falls into
plantar flexion (figure 6.6*a*), and even with the application of a strong passive stretch,
the ankle may only reach 90 degrees of dorsiflexion (figure 6.6*b*).

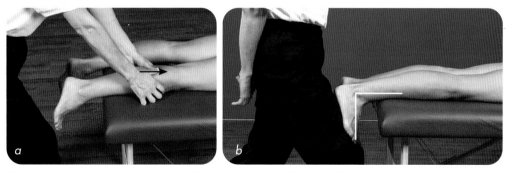

Figure 6.6   *(a)* At rest, the ankle falls into plantar flexion; *(b)* passive stretching may
increase the range of motion to around 90 degrees.

The calf muscles are extremely strong, allowing us to raise up onto our tiptoes. Therefore, active stretches are one of the best ways to increase dorsiflexion past 90 degrees; your client can use their own body weight to increase the angle of the ankle by placing a block beneath the toes (figure 6.7a) or standing with one leg behind the body (figure 6.7b). Notice that in each of these stretches, the angle of the ankle is less than 90 degrees.

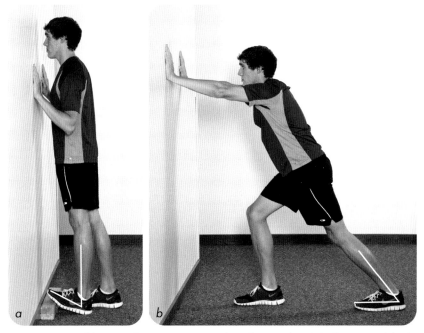

Figure 6.7 Active ankle stretches to improve dorsiflexion by *(a)* placing a block beneath the toes or *(b)* putting the leg behind the body.

TIP

It is important to include stretches to the toes, especially the flexor muscles, because the long tendons of these muscles cross the ankle joint and therefore affect the ankle's range of motion. Please see the discussion on plantar fasciitis and stiff feet in the next section for how to do this.

Plantar Fasciitis and Stiff Feet

Much more research is needed to understand the exact aetiology of plantar fasciitis. Excessive strain may lead to microtrauma, inflammation and degeneration. It is unlikely that this condition results purely from inflammation of the fascia, and the term *fasciosis* may be more appropriate. The plantar fascia is consistent with the fascia of the calf via the calcaneus, and massaging and stretching the tissues of one (i.e., of the foot or of the calf) is likely to improve extensibility in tissues of the other area. This in turn could theoretically reduce strain on the plantar fascia.

Massage

All of the massage techniques described in the section on tight calf muscles in chapter 5 and the hamstrings in chapter 4 are appropriate. Massaging the sole of the foot by using your fingers to spread and stretch the soft tissues of the metatarsal heads is also helpful provided that it is not painful. Stroking the foot with the fist (figure 6.8) can be soothing, but in many people, the sole is very sore, and you may need to restrict your massage to the calf alone.

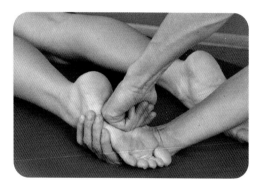

Figure 6.8 Massaging the sole of the foot using gentle strokes with the fist.

Trigger Point Release

In a study of 100 patients with plantar fasciopathy, Thummar, Rajaseker and Anumasa (2020) found that trigger points in the medial gastrocnemius and quadratus plantae muscles were strongly associated with plantar fasciitis, as were trigger points in the soleus, tibialis posterior, adductor hallucis and adductor longus muscles. Arif and colleagues (2018) applied trigger point release to the gastrocnemius and soleus muscles and the plantar fascia in a group of 42 patients diagnosed with plantar fasciitis. The patients were treated three times a week for 4 weeks. A plantar fasciitis pain scale questionnaire was used before and after intervention. This scale measured pain on awakening, when standing, walking or running and when ascending and descending stairs. The intensity of the pain when walking was significantly reduced after the treatment. There was also a reduction in pain when standing and stair climbing.

Stretching

In a clinical consensus statement, the American College of Foot and Ankle Surgeons stated that stretching is a safe and effective treatment for plantar fasciitis (Schneider et al. 2018). Due to the connections of the fascia from the posterior thigh to the calf and to the foot, it is always useful to include hamstring and calf stretches when treating this condition. All the stretches shown for the treatment of tight hamstrings in chapter 4 and a tight calf in chapter 5 could be used. The plantar fascia covers part of the sole of the foot, and stretching the toes into extension will tense this fascia (figure 6.9).

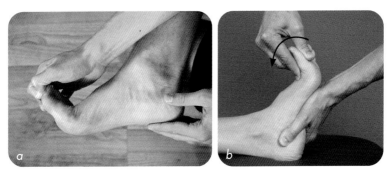

Figure 6.9 Extension of the toes, (a) actively and (b) passively, helps to tense the plantar fascia.

In figure 6.10, the client has the benefit of being able to use body weight to help facilitate the stretch, but for some clients and in acute stages of plantar fasciitis, this may be too uncomfortable. A third form of active stretching is for the client to slowly roll the foot over a hard ball, such as a golf ball (figure 6.11). This stretches small sections of the fascia, which may have an overall beneficial effect. If you decide to recommend this stretch, make sure the client does not attempt to stand on the golf ball but instead performs the stretch whilst sitting and gently rolls the foot over the ball.

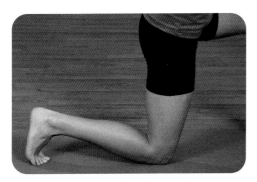

Figure 6.10 Using body weight to extend the toes and stretch the sole of the foot.

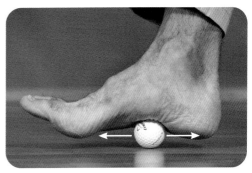

Figure 6.11 Using a ball to microstretch small areas of the sole of the foot.

Specialist Referrals

In the case of a stiff foot, referral to a physiotherapist, osteopath or chiropractor may be helpful, because these professionals can use techniques to mobilise individual bones of the foot and toes.

Pes Planus (Flatfoot)

People with pes planus experience pain in the foot, often in the region of the posterior tibial tendon, and struggle to perform a single-leg heel raise. If flatfoot is due to structural abnormality and is rigid, hands-on therapy is ineffective. The main focus of your treatment for flexible flatfoot is on the prevention of excessive pronation when the foot is loaded, and this is achieved by controlling valgus (eversion) of the calcaneus (Levangie and Norkin 2001). Please refer to the pes valgus section of this chapter. Be aware that changes made to the position of bones of the foot affect not only the lower limb but the entire kinetic chain throughout the body. Your client may experience either relief from or an exacerbation of symptoms elsewhere as a result of treatments to the foot.

Massage

Massage to the foot and leg, using any technique, may be helpful in alleviating pain.

Stretching

All of the gastrocnemius and soleus stretches shown in chapter 5 for the treatment of a tight calf are useful, as are figures 6.9, 6.10 and 6.11.

Strengthening

Popularly known as foot gymnastics, foot dexterity exercises are sometimes used to help strengthen the intrinsic muscles of the foot. However, these have not been shown to be effective over and above general exercise (Hartmann et al. 2009). Please see chapter 9 for more information.

Manual Therapist

Referral to a manual therapist (e.g., a physical therapist, osteopath or chiropractor) who can mobilise the bones of the foot and toes may be helpful, because this mobilisation will assist with the overall flexibility of the foot.

The American College of Foot and Ankle Surgeons (2023a) recommend a reduction in body weight in patients who are overweight, because putting too much weight on the foot arches may aggravate symptoms. Therefore, where appropriate, refer your client to a dietician.

You might also refer your client to a podiatrist, who may be able to offer advice on the use of orthotics. There is moderate evidence that orthotics may improve walking function and reduce energy used when walking but only low-level evidence that they improve pain, reduce rearfoot eversion, alter loading and impact forces and reduce rearfoot inversion movements (Banwell, Mackintosh, and Thewlis 2014). If the flatfoot is the result of dysfunction in the tibialis posterior, wearing flat, lace-up footwear that can accommodate orthosis may help (Kohls-Gatzoulis et al. 2004).

Pes Cavus (High Arches)

In the pes cavus foot posture, stress is placed on the ball of the foot and the heel. The extra weight placed on the metatarsal heads of the toes can cause pain, and people with this condition may report feeling unbalanced. If pes cavus is the result of a neurological condition, hands-on therapy will be ineffective. Some studies have shown that there is no evidence for the effectiveness of any treatments other than orthotics for the pes cavus posture (Burns et al. 2007). Be aware that changes made to the position of bones of the foot affect not only the lower limb but the entire kinetic chain throughout the body. Your client may have either relief from or an exacerbation of symptoms elsewhere as a result of treatments to the foot.

Massage

Although stretching of the plantar fascia with massage and passive dorsiflexion of the toes may provide some pain relief, there is little evidence to show that it affects pes cavus foot posture.

Stretching

Stretching of the gastrocnemius has been advocated as a useful non-surgical intervention for pes cavus (Manoli and Graham 2005). Please refer to the gastrocnemius and soleus stretches shown the section on tight calf muscles in chapter 5.

Strengthening

People with pes cavus foot posture are likely to benefit from balance training. This will not change the posture of the foot but will improve balance, reducing the likelihood of injury from, for example, sprains. For more information on balance training, please see chapter 9.

Podiatry

Consider referring your client to a podiatrist. Orthotics, shoe modifications and bracing may be helpful (American College of Foot and Ankle Surgeons 2023b). Custom-made orthotics have been shown to provide significant benefit (Burns et al. 2007). The goal of these is to realign the hindfoot and offload the lateral side of the foot.

Pes Valgus (Pronated Foot)

You learned in chapter 1 that in the pes valgus posture, there is eversion of the heel away from the midline position. The consequence of this is that the foot pronates and there is loss of the medial longitudinal arch. This causes an increase in compression of the soft tissues of the lateral side of the ankle and tensing of the tissues on the medial side of the ankle.

Massage

Massage to shortened muscles (the fibular muscles and possibly the gastrocnemius and soleus) may reduce tension that results from this foot posture, but it will not affect the underlying foot structure.

Soft Tissue Release

Soft tissue release could be used to release tension in the fibular muscles, perhaps with your client in a side-lying position (figure 6.12). First, ask your client to evert their ankle; then, apply static pressure to the lateral side of the calf and maintain this pressure as you ask your client to invert their ankle. Work from proximal to distal. You may need to experiment with positioning the client's leg on a bolster to facilitate movement of the ankle

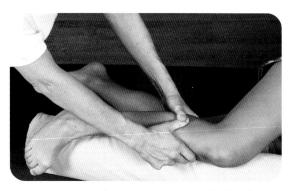

Figure 6.12 Soft tissue release to the fibular muscles.

that would otherwise be restricted by the treatment couch. Take care not to compress the peroneal nerve, which passes around the head of the fibula.

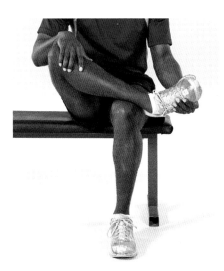

Stretching

Active stretching may reduce tension in the fibular muscles, which are evertor muscles (figure 6.13). Also stretch the muscles of the hip and thigh, such as the hamstrings and adductors, if these are found to be tight. For stretches to these muscles, please see the sections on tight hip adductors in chapter 3 and tight hamstrings in chapter 4.

Figure 6.13 An active stretch of the fibular muscles.

Taping

Taping is a popular intervention for the treatment of pes valgus. However, an experiment by Luque-Suarez and colleagues (2014) to see whether the application of Kinesio Tape helped correct excessive foot pronation found that it did not. Another study found that taping to correct pronation during walking and jogging was effective (Vicenzino et al. 2005).

Strengthening

Useful exercises are those for the ankle invertor muscles (chapter 9) and weakened muscles of the hip, such as the gluteal muscles (chapter 7). These are likely to help with overall strength and balance but are unlikely to change underlying foot posture.

Myofascial Release and Podiatry

Use myofascial release for the whole lateral side of the lower limb.

TIP

Advise your client to avoid resting the feet around chair legs when sitting, because this pushes the feet into eversion (figure 6.14).

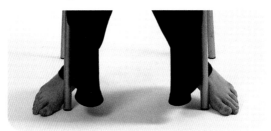

Figure 6.14   A seated foot posture to avoid.

Courtesy of Emma Kelly Photography.

Refer your client to a podiatrist. The use of orthotics to control the amount of prona-tion (for example, during the stance phase of gait) has profound effects on pain and dysfunction in the lower extremity (Donatelli 1987).

Pes Varus (Supinated Foot)

In the supinated foot posture, the heel bone moves towards the midline, accentuating the medial longitudinal arch. In contrast to the pes valgus foot posture, there is increased pressure on the medial side of the ankle, and the lateral side of the ankle is tensed.

Massage

Massage and stretch shortened tissues (in this case, on the plantar surface of the foot), focusing on the medial side and the medial aspect of the ankle and taking care not to apply too much pressure. Positioning your client in a side-lying position can be useful for applying massage to the medial side of the leg (figure 6.15a), and using a towel (figure 6.15b) or your thigh (figure 6.15c) can help you access and stretch tissues on the medial side of the ankle.

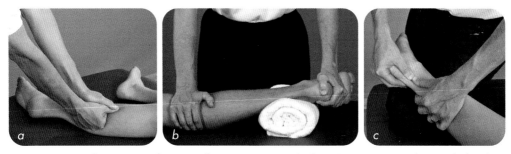

Figure 6.15 Therapist techniques for pes varus include (a) massage to the medial side of the leg, perhaps positioning the client with the medial side of the ankle uppermost using (b) a towel or (c) your thigh.

Stretching

Show your client how to stretch the medial side of the foot and foot invertors by placing a small, folded towel beneath the lateral side of the foot (figure 6.16a). Active (figure 6.16b) and passive (figure 6.16c) stretching of the flexor hallucis longus is also useful.

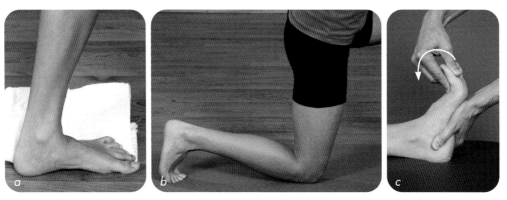

Figure 6.16 Stretches for pes varus include (a) actively stretching the ankle invertor muscles by standing on a towel and (b) actively and (c) passively stretching the flexor hallucis longus.

Strengthening

Strengthen ankle evertors. Please see chapter 9 for more information.

Podiatry

Refer your client to a podiatrist. The use of orthotics to control the amount of supination during the stance phase of gait, for example, has profound effects on pain and dysfunction in the lower extremity (Donatelli 1987). The lateral side of the foot can be elevated with orthotics, but it is not clear whether this has a function in altering foot and ankle posture. Use of lateral wedge orthotics has been found to reduce symptoms in patients with medial compartment osteoarthritis at the knee (Malvankar et al. 2012), so it may alter lower limb posture. One of the challenges with the pes varus posture is that orthotics designed to correct foot supination can aggravate genu valgum where this is a corresponding posture.

Quick Questions

1. Why is it necessary to educate your client with regards to the importance of rehabilitation after an ankle sprain?

2. When working with someone who had their ankle immobilised after a fracture, which joints in addition to the ankle should be mobilised and stretched?

3. Why is it useful to stretch the ankle joint to more than 90 degrees of dorsiflexion as part of treatment for a stiff ankle?

4. Which part of the ankle is compressed in the pes valgus foot posture?

5. On which side of the leg, ankle and foot should you focus when applying massage in the treatment of the pes varus foot posture?

Lower Limb Strengthening Exercises

Part III provides examples of strengthening exercises used in the treatment of the lower limb conditions described in this book. Chapter 7 focuses on hip strengthening, chapter 8 on knee strengthening and chapter 9 on strengthening of the feet and ankles. The rationale behind providing a separate part on strengthening exercises is that you may be a soft tissue therapist and unfamiliar with strengthening protocols, because these are not usually covered in massage and other soft tissue training courses. If you have a background in fitness and rehabilitation, then you may already be familiar with the material in these chapters. In the author's experience, only a minority of soft tissue therapists work alongside fitness professionals or clinicians who can provide strengthening programmes, and they may be unaware of simple exercises that are a useful adjunct to soft tissue treatment.

The purpose of this part of the book is not to teach you to become a fitness professional. You do not necessarily need to provide the exercises described here to your client; simply knowing which exercises are used – and, importantly, why they are used – can be extremely helpful in supporting your client to recover from or manage their condition. Adherence to exercise programmes is known to be poor, and in itself, a discussion around adherence might improve compliance and therefore hasten recovery.

Testing Lower Limb Strength

Each chapter in part III describes how to identify whether a person lacks strength in a particular muscle group. The strength tests described rely either on the client attempting a movement and informing you as to whether they perceive a strength deficit between the left and right limbs or your providing manual resistance to a movement and forming your own opinion as to whether there is a deficit. Ultimately, the goal of a strength training programme is to help a person to regain everyday function, as far as is possible. It could be argued that functional ability is more important to measure over and above the isolated strength of a particular muscle group. Therefore, you can also use the examples of functional strengthening exercises as measures of strength.

Strengthening Exercise Types

There are many different types of lower limb strengthening exercises, such as exercises to develop pure strength and muscle bulk, where a person performs a single repetition involving the maximum weight they can lift. These are typically used by powerlifters and bodybuilders, who might perform a single knee extension using a knee extension machine. Another type of lower limb strengthening exercise is endurance training, where the focus is to build stamina in a group of muscles by repeating the same exercise, perhaps in three sets of 8 or 12 repetitions, with a minute's rest between sets. These kinds of lower limb exercises are typically performed by people whose sporting activity relies on lower limb endurance, such as footballers or runners. The exercises in this part of the book have been selected to facilitate early recovery from a lower limb problem, and they fall more into the category of the endurance required to regain function and a return to everyday activities.

Regaining Function After an Injury

Keep in mind tasks that must be done in everyday life and that your client may be struggling with, such as getting out of bed, standing, walking, sitting down onto a chair, getting up out of a chair, getting washed and getting dressed. These are the activities that we ultimately wish to facilitate through the use of strength and balance exercises, and the exercises provided in chapters 7, 8 and 9 have this aim in mind. However, there will be many clients who cannot yet bear weight through a joint, so standing and walking are not possible. This is especially true after a fracture to the lower limb or a severe sprain; weight bearing needs to be avoided, but it is still possible to perform other, safe exercises.

Non-Functional Exercises Versus Functional Exercises

Many clinicians dislike non-functional exercises. Range-of-motion exercises – such as actively bending and straightening the knee in isolation, circling the ankle or performing repeated abduction of the hip in a side-lying position – are examples of non-functional exercises. Isolated movements such as these do not replicate what we need to do with our lower limbs in real life – bearing weight through them, walking, stepping up and down off a pathway, using stairs, squatting down, driving and so on. However, there is a place for non-functional exercises as well as functional exercises, such as when a person cannot perform their usual functions but can perform some other movement. A typical example is in the case of a severe ankle sprain. In such cases, a person cannot bear weight through the foot or ankle because to do so in the early stages of recovery would be injurious; they may be unable to bear weight and require crutches to ambulate. It is not possible for them to replicate certain activities of daily life, such as normal walking. Without engagement in a recovery programme, the muscles of the lower limb will atrophy and lose strength because they are not being used. Many clients recovering from a severe ankle sprain complain of pain in the low back or opposite limb due to an altered gait pattern and overcompensating with use of their other leg. In this example, a useful way to maintain strength in the lower limb is with hip, thigh and knee strengthening.

The exercises that have been selected for inclusion in this part of the book are safe and effective; they rely only on the use of a client's body weight or a resistance band. Resistance bands are available in different degrees of resistance (light, medium and heavy) and are inexpensive, lightweight and easy to store. The value of the exercises presented in part III is that they can be performed at home; to help a person recover or manage a lower limb condition, it is not necessary to have access to a gymnasium or to exercise weights. Stretches are not included in this part of the book; examples of stretches are found in chapters 3, 4, 5 and 6, alongside the conditions for which they may be useful.

Balance Exercises

After an injury to the lower limb, the ability to balance is almost always compromised. The longer someone has been inactive, the poorer their balance is likely to be. Balance exercises are therefore extremely important and are included in chapter 9. You may have seen or heard of people standing on a 'wobble' board as part of their recovery from an ankle sprain. Instructions for using wobble boards and similar devices are not included, as these devices should be used towards the end of the rehabilitation phase and a mistake is to use them too soon, risking reinjury. Instead, simple balance exercises are provided and are likely to be essential for the recovery from most lower limb conditions.

The types of balance exercises included in chapter 9 are those that involve weight bearing through both legs whilst transferring weight from one leg to the other using various foot positions. In addition, there are explanations of how to make simple single-leg balancing exercises more challenging and thus safely facilitate an improvement in balance. The value of the exercises provided in this chapter is that they can be used early on in the rehabilitation programme.

Exercise Positions and Repetitions

Exercises are included for sitting, supine, prone and side-lying positions, to be used where weight-bearing is not yet possible. The position in which exercises are performed and the number of repetitions performed for each exercise depend on many different factors: your client's tolerance to each position, the stage of their recovery and their general health and fitness needs, for example. Most important is the need to establish the ultimate goal you and the client are aiming for. This is likely to change over time.

A typical endurance programme might start with two or three sets each of 5 to 7 repetitions, increasing to 12 repetitions. Although many therapists prescribe such an exercise programme to be performed daily or even up to three times daily, in the author's experience, this can be detrimental and cause fatigue and muscle soreness. This then reduces the client's motivation to continue with the programme. It is better to perform an exercise well, using perhaps a smaller number of sets or repetitions, than to perform an exercise poorly, which tends to happen when people become fatigued or bored.

Exercise Progression

Where possible, the exercises have been presented in order from those that require the least strength to those that require more strength. However, what one person finds challenging, another might find easy. Once a person is used to a certain exercise, it is beneficial to change to one requiring more strength. By contrast, if exercises are too challenging to perform, there is a risk that the person will become demotivated or reinjure themselves, which is why it is important for your client to set realistic goals. The exercises provided in this part of the book are basic and focus on the early stages of recovery. The exercises are not designed to help someone return to recreational or competitive sport, for which more intensive and highly varied rehabilitation programmes are needed and supervision by an exercise specialist is recommended.

Improving Exercise Plan Adherence

People quickly become bored with rehabilitation exercise, and their adherence may lessen. This lack of adherence delays recovery. Most people want to return to their everyday activities. Your challenge is therefore to help a client regain usual function as soon as possible and to encourage adherence to an exercise plan as soon as it is safe and practical. Table III.1 shows some of the reasons for non-adherence to an exercise plan and gives suggestions for how to overcome these.

Note: Special thanks to Tim Allardyce from rehabmypatient.com for permission to reproduce the strengthening exercises in chapters 7, 8 and 9. Rehab My Patient is an online resource containing thousands of exercises, not just the small selection of strengthening exercises that have been selected for inclusion in this book.

Table III.1   Why Exercise Plans Fail and Solutions to Overcome This

Reasons for exercise plan failure	Solutions
A common misconception is that recovery requires 'hands-on' treatment or that intervention by someone else is needed to 'fix' a condition. Therapists may often have heard someone complain that 'they never even touched me. They just gave me a sheet of exercises'.	Clients need to be educated with regards to the value of exercise, because in most cases, the reason certain exercises have been prescribed is that they are the most likely to facilitate recovery.
Clients may fail to understand the purpose of an exercise and therefore do not value it.	The rationale for the exercise needs to be clearly explained. For example, the rationale for the stretches described in previous chapters is to improve range of motion in a joint, aid flexibility and help manage symptoms, whereas the exercises described in chapters 7, 8 and 9 are designed to improve muscle and joint strength and balance. It is important to explain the rationale for an exercise that involves strengthening a different body part to that which is affected. For example, it is important to explain to someone recovering from a knee or ankle issue that the gluteal 'bridge' exercise helps strengthen the buttock muscles and that this is important for hip strength and stability, which is compromised during periods of immobilisation, whether due to injury or illness.
Providing too many of the same exercises without variety quickly becomes boring.	Provide safe alternatives to each exercise. The way to do this effectively is careful monitoring of the client's improvement and changing an exercise to become slightly more challenging once they are ready to progress. This could be done by changing the exercise itself or by changing the position in which it is performed.
The exercise is too difficult or too hard. A common mistake when providing an exercise programme is to give every client with the same injury the same programme.	Programmes need to be individually tailored so that they are challenging enough to be slightly effortful but not so challenging that they are impossible.
Clients may believe that all exercise should be pain free.	Exercises should not cause excruciating pain, but some discomfort is almost always experienced during or after exercise, as this is a normal part of the strengthening process. Educating your clients in this regard is helpful.

(continued)

Table III.1 Why Exercise Plans Fail and Solutions to Overcome This *(continued)*

Reasons for exercise plan failure	Solutions
Too many or too few exercises may have been provided. Some clients become overwhelmed if they are given too many exercises. If it takes a long time to complete a series of exercises, adherence can be affected. Conversely, if too few exercises are provided, some clients, especially those used to physical activity, quickly become bored and frustrated at what they perceive to be slow progress.	It is important to tailor a programme to each client. For example, someone who tires easily due to an underlying condition might benefit more from a smaller number of sets and repetitions than someone who does not fatigue quickly. Someone who is easily bored may need to be provided with a greater variety of exercises or a programme where the exercises are varied on alternate days.
Clients may fail to improve due to poor technique. A lack of attention can lead to repetition of a poor movement pattern, which in itself can be detrimental to overall recovery.	All exercises should be completed with care and concentration. The exercises provided in this part of the book are very simple and do not require a great deal of explanation, but where possible, clients should be observed performing their exercises and be given constructive feedback.
Clients fail to see improvement despite adherence.	To regain strength, it is important to progress exercises appropriately, eventually progressing to functional exercises. Failure to do this risks that a client will become very good at one or a few specific exercises but will never progress beyond these. Use of an exercise diary can be invaluable.

Hips

Learning Outcomes

After reading this chapter, you should be able to do the following:

- Demonstrate simple tests to determine the strength of the hip extensors, hip abductors, hip adductors and hip flexors.
- Show examples of hip strengthening exercises.
- Teach hip strengthening exercises in prone, supine, side-lying, sitting and standing positions.
- Explain how to make any of the exercises in this chapter harder or easier.
- List examples of functional hip exercises.
- Identify which hip strengthening exercises may also be appropriate for common conditions affecting the thigh, knee, ankle and foot.

This chapter focuses entirely on exercises to strengthen the hip and thigh region. These exercises are suitable in the treatment of the conditions discussed in chapter 3 (trigger points in the gluteal muscles, piriformis syndrome, tight hip adductors, tight hip flexors and groin strain). Many of the exercises in this chapter are also useful in the treatment of knee, ankle or foot problems, for which strength and stability in the hip are essential to recovery or general maintenance of everyday function.

Testing the Strength of the Hip Muscles

When treating people with any of the lower limb conditions described in this book, you are encouraged to test the strength of the hip muscles. Hip muscle weakness is extremely common after immobilisation, even if the injury or condition affects the knee or ankle. This chapter describes how to test the strength of the hip extensors, flexors, abductors and adductors. The need for isolated hip rotation, whether internal or external, is rare; therefore, tests for the strength of those isolated movements are not included.

Hip Extensors

Identifying Weakness in the Hip Extensors

One of the simplest ways to test the strength of the hip extensors is to ask your client to perform a 'bridge' exercise (figure 7.1a). If they can do this, have them repeat the test using one leg at a time and compare both sides (figure 7.1b). Look for three things to determine weakness. First, how easy does this appear for the client? Second, is the client able to keep the pelvis level and parallel to the floor or plinth, indicating strength, or does the side being lifted drop down, indicating weakness? Third, is there any shaking? Get the client's feedback as to whether it feels easier to lift the left or the right leg. Obviously, this test is unsuitable for a client who cannot bear weight through their knee or ankle, in which case, you could ask them to attempt hip extension using the prone (figure 7.1c) or side-lying positions (figure 7.1d), getting their feedback as to which hip feels weaker. The tests for hip extensor strength can also be used as strengthening exercises.

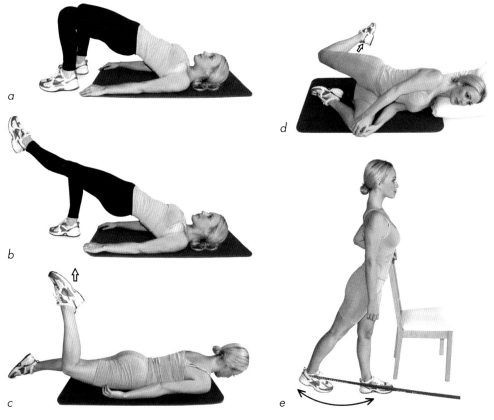

Figure 7.1 Testing and strengthening the hip extensors in (a, b) supine, (c) prone, (d) side-lying and (e) standing positions.

Courtesy of Tim Allardyce, Rehabmypatient.com.

Hip Extensor Strengthening

Hip extensor strengthening is part of a general gluteal strengthening programme and is useful whenever there is weakness in the extensors, as may occur when the hip adductor muscles are tight, after a person has sustained a groin strain or when a person has piriformis syndrome. Strengthening is particularly helpful if a person has tightness in the hip flexors, because strengthening of the hip extensor muscles will reduce tone in the hip flexors.

Because the hamstrings are hip extensors in addition to being flexors of the knee, there may be hip extensor weakness after a hamstring strain or when there is tightness in the hamstrings. Sensations of tightness in a muscle could indicate that the hamstring muscles are shortened, and when this occurs, this muscle group is often weak.

TIP

Note that hip extension is only one test for weakness in the hamstrings, and knee flexor strength should also be tested. Please see chapter 8 for instructions.

Hip extension may be performed in supine, prone and standing positions. One of the easiest ways to strengthen hip extensors is in the supine position by simply lifting the buttocks from the floor (see figure 7.1a) without arching the back. To make this more challenging, one leg can be extended whilst lifting the hips using the other leg (see figure 7.1b). The aim of the one-leg position is to keep the pelvis level and to prevent it from dropping towards the floor or plinth.

TIP

To make the exercise shown in figure 7.1b more difficult, the hips can be lifted whilst the arms are folded across the chest. Even harder still is to use the extended leg to draw circles in the air, thus adding the need for stabilisation of the pelvis and therefore greater strength. Alternatively, instead of extending the leg, the foot could be rested on the knee of the supporting leg, adding weight.

Hip extension in the prone position (see figure 7.1c) requires lifting the leg against gravity, which necessitates more strength than performing this exercise in the side-lying position (see figure 7.1d). The side-lying position is less stable, but it may be useful if the client has muscle weakness.

TIP

When teaching the prone version of hip extensor strengthening, a tip is to ask your client to try to 'place a footprint on the ceiling'.

Hip extension can also be performed when standing (see figure 7.1e). Using a resistance band increases the difficulty. This is a more functional activity than performing the exercises lying down, but it requires strength and stability of the opposite leg, and the client needs to keep their chest upright and avoid bending at the waist.

Active Hip Contraction

Some clients cannot perform movements of the hip because, for instance, they have knee or ankle pain or instability. An example might be when someone has sustained an injury to the knee or ankle that requires immobilisation in a cast or brace and ambulation is severely restricted. In this example, contraction of the buttock muscles, whether lying or sitting, will help minimise loss of strength in the gluteal muscles.

Making Hip Extension More Functional

Many functional activities, such as sit-to-stand movements and stair climbing, rely on strength in the gluteal muscles, and these activities can therefore be used as part of the rehabilitation programme. Simply standing up from a sitting position (figure 7.2a) or stepping up as when using stairs (figure 7.2b) requires strength in the gluteal muscles. These activities could therefore be included in a hip extensor strengthening programme. Because they also require strength in the quadriceps muscles, these exercises are often used as part of the rehabilitation programme for clients with knee problems too.

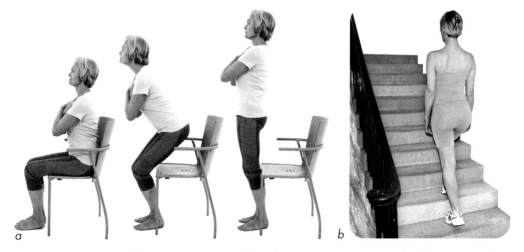

Figure 7.2 Functional exercises to strengthen the hip extensors include *(a)* sit-to-stand movements and *(b)* stair climbing.

Courtesy of Tim Allardyce, Rehabmypatient.com.

To make a sit-to-stand exercise easier, the client could use their hands to press up out of the chair. To make the exercise more difficult, the client could place more weight through their affected leg. To make it harder still, they could practise sit-to-stand exercises using one leg only.

Note that the exercises in figure 7.2 are different to those in figure 7.1, and not only in that they are more functional. Compare the position of the hip in figures 7.1 and 7.2. Notice how in figure 7.2, the hip starts in hip flexion and ends in a neutral position, whereas in figure 7.1, the hip starts in a neutral position and ends up in extension. This is why a variety of different exercises is almost always advocated, because different types of exercises work the muscles of extension in different ways and therefore provide optimal strengthening.

Hip Abductors

Identifying Weakness in the Hip Abductors

A simple test of strength in the hip abductors is to ask your client to sit (or lie supine) with their knees together and the hips and knees flexed and to abduct against resistance you provide using your hands or against the resistance of an exercise band (figure 7.3a), giving you feedback as to which side feels weaker. Another useful test is the exercise shown in figure 7.3b. If there is weakness, the client will struggle to abduct the leg, but note that straight-leg abduction in the supine position can also be hampered by resistance from the surface on which the client is lying, such as a towel or bedding. The exercises in figures 7.3c and 7.3d both require more strength as the leg (7.3c) or pelvis (7.3d) is lifted against gravity. These are useful tests for people with considerable pre-existing hip strength, such as those engaged in regular sporting activities. Where there is weakness in the hip abductors, the client will struggle to maintain the position of the abducted leg or to keep the pelvis lifted, depending on which test is used. The strength of the hip abductors can also be tested in the standing position (figure 7.3e).

Hip Abductor Strengthening

Hip abduction occurs when taking the leg out to the side, such as when stepping sideways when walking. Weakness occurs with disuse of the limb after immobilisation or injury, but weakness in the gluteus medius may also be present in people who are physically active.

One of the most stable positions in which to perform strengthening of the hip abductors is the supine position. In this exercise, the client simply abducts their hips. Usually, what limits this movement is tightness in the muscles of the groin, not weakness in the abductor muscles. Therefore, to make this exercise more effective, a stretchy exercise band can be used (figure 7.3a).

TIP

If a person struggles with the exercise in figure 7.3a, they could perform it without the exercise band. Some people prefer to perform the exercise seated, with or without a band.

The supine straight-leg abduction (figure 7.3b) and side-lying with knees flexed (figure 7.3d) positions can also be adopted to strengthen the hip abductors.

TIP

Although the supine position looks relatively easy, the lower limb is extremely heavy, and to abduct the entire lower limb requires simultaneous hip flexion to raise the limb slightly from the floor. This can be challenging for people with weak abdominal muscles or who have conditions affecting the low back. Flexing the hip and knee on the side opposite to the limb being exercised can help make this position more comfortable, because this brings about a posterior tilt in the pelvis, reducing lumbar extension. To make the exercise easier, the leg could be moved against a slippery surface, such as plastic sheeting.

Hip abduction can also be performed in the standing position (figure 7.3e), requiring stability in the supporting leg and avoidance of leaning over to one side, away from the hip being strengthened.

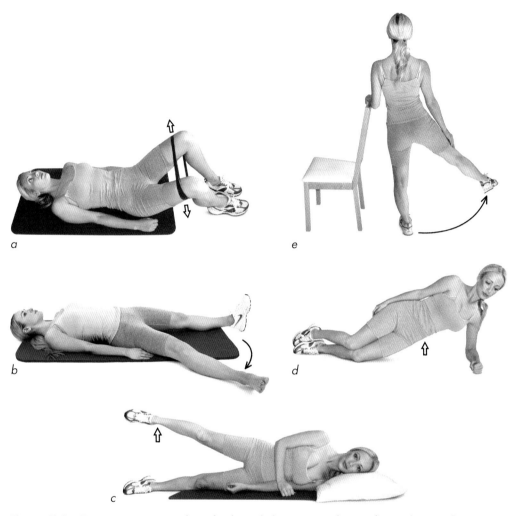

Figure 7.3 Exercises to strengthen the hip abductors can be performed in (a, b) supine, (c, d) side-lying and (e) standing positions.

Courtesy of Tim Allardyce, Rehabmypatient.com.

When performing hip abduction in the standing position, placing a resistance band above the knees makes the exercise more difficult, and placing the band around the ankles makes it even more challenging. Using the band around the ankles is not appropriate for people with knee issues, because greater strain is placed on the knee to abduct the hip against resistance in this way.

Abduction of the lower limb in a side-lying position (figure 7.3c) is one of the most challenging exercises, because it requires lifting the entire lower limb against gravity. This is therefore a good exercise to aim for once other positions have been tried. In this position, it is important to keep the body straight and to avoid leaning forwards or backwards.

To make the exercise in figure 7.3c more difficult, a resistance band can be placed around the thighs. To increase resistance even further, the band can be placed around the ankles. Again, care is needed when working with people who have knee issues, because a band around the ankles adds strain to the lateral aspect of the knee. In someone with healthy knees, using a band should cause no problems, but it is useful to be aware of the risk. An alternative to using a band to make the exercise more difficult is to perform movements of the abducted leg, such as small circles in the air, thus compromising stability and requiring greater strength to balance the body.

Making Hip Abduction More Functional

Two very useful exercises can make hip abduction more functional. The first is simple sidestepping, which exercises both the hip abductors and the hip adductors. This exercise could involve sidestepping across the room, for example. In early stages of rehabilitation or when working with someone with balance issues, sidestepping can be done with a support (figure 7.4a). Another useful exercise is stepping sideways up and onto a step (figure 7.4b). This action requires hip flexion to lift the leg, then contraction of the hip abductors and extensors to lift the body weight to the step height. This exercise could easily be performed on the bottom step of a staircase at home.

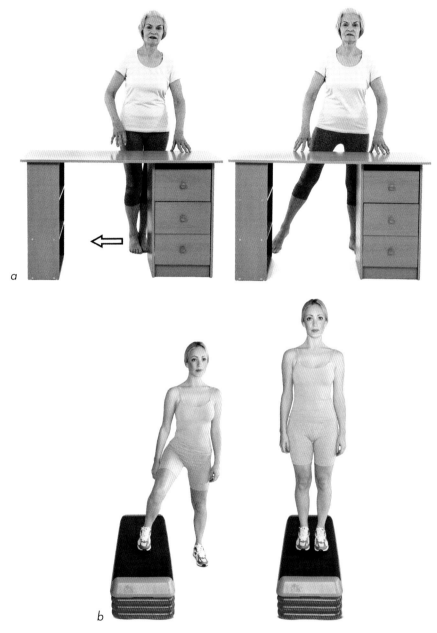

Figure 7.4 Making hip abduction exercises more functional includes *(a)* sidestepping and *(b)* side step-ups.

Courtesy of Tim Allardyce, Rehabmypatient.com.

Hip Adductors

Identifying Weakness in the Hip Adductors

In the supine position, weakness in the hip adductors can be tested by asking the client to rest with both legs abducted in a frog-type position and to then try to bring their knees together (figure 7.5a). This has the advantage of enabling you to compare one hip with the other. Look for any shaking, indicating weakness, and ask the client whether they noticed that it was easier to adduct one hip compared to the other. If the client has an issue affecting movement of the non-affected hip, the test can be performed unilaterally (figure 7.5b). The disadvantage of this is that you cannot compare the strength of that hip with the opposite side and therefore do not know whether the strength at the time of testing is normal for your client. You can teach your client how to compare the strength of their hips using a sitting position (figure 7.5c). The side-lying position (figure 7.5d) is perhaps the most challenging for hip strength, because it requires the client to adduct their hip against gravity. The degree of reported effort, combined with how far the leg can be lifted or for how long the lift can be sustained, is a helpful indication of the strength of the hip adductors.

Hip Adductor Strengthening

Strengthening of hip adductors is important after a groin strain, especially when this is chronic. Strains of the adductor muscles can take up to 16 weeks to heal, depending on their severity, and it is important to start a strengthening programme as soon as possible.

A simple strengthening exercise is for the client to attempt to squeeze the knees together. This isometric exercise is good because it can be performed seated, supine or even in a side-lying position. One of the easiest hip adduction strengthening exercises is performed in the supine position. Many people have tight hip adductors and will not be able to let their knees fall open to touch the ground. That is OK, because this exercise is not about hip flexibility but strength. The client either brings their knees back together bilaterally (figure 7.5a) or unilaterally (figure 7.5b). Clients often feel more balanced performing the exercise with both legs simultaneously, but this is not essential.

TIP

An easy way to make the exercises in figures 7.5a and 7.5b more challenging is for the client to start to bring the knees (or knee) back to the midline but to hold the leg midway between the fullest abduction and fullest adduction. This requires the adductors to hold the weight of the leg without moving, and the duration of the hold could be used to determine improvements in muscle endurance.

Strengthening could also be performed in the seated position, where the client sits with the hips abducted to begin and then tries to bring the knees together. To increase the difficulty, the client could apply resistance by pressing their hands against their knees (figure 7.5c). Finally, a very simple way to make hip adduction more challenging is to lift the whole lower limb from the floor, as in figure 7.5d.

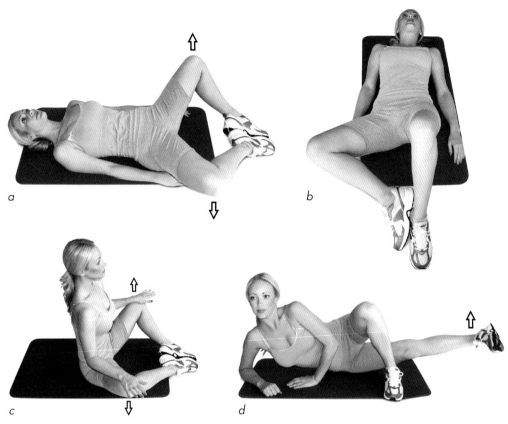

Figure 7.5 Hip adductor strengthening can be performed in the *(a, b)* supine, *(c)* seated or *(d)* side-lying positions.

Courtesy of Tim Allardyce, Rehabmypatient.com.

Making Hip Adduction More Functional

You may not realise it, but whenever you walk, your hip adductors contract to help keep you walking in a straight line. Therefore, walking is an excellent part of hip rehabilitation. The exercises shown in figure 7.4 are also useful because they require action in both the hip abductors and adductors.

HIP FLEXORS

Hip Flexors

Identifying Weakness in the Hip Flexors

With your client seated, ask them to lift one knee at a time, with resistance (figure 7.6a), and to let you know whether it feels more difficult to lift one leg or the other. Another way to test this is whilst you provide resistance with your hand (as in the seated position) or with your client lying supine (figure 7.6b). Having your client attempt a hip flexion, whether standing (figure 7.6c) or lying down (figure 7.6d), is another way to determine the strength of the hip flexors and has the advantage of being more objective, because you can observe the distance the leg can be lifted.

Hip Flexor Strengthening

Pressing the knee against resistance (figure 7.6a) can be used as an isometric strengthening exercise.

TIP

To make hip strengthening easier, the client could perform this exercise in the supine position (figure 7.6b). In this position, they are not lifting the knee against gravity, so this is useful in the early stages of rehabilitation.

Lifting the leg against gravity can be performed standing (figure 7.6c) or lying down (figure 7.6d). When the knee is extended, lifting the leg requires more strength, so performing a straight-leg raise in the supine (figure 7.6d) position is more difficult than when the knee is flexed (figure 7.6b).

Many people have shortened hip flexors that feel 'tight' on attempting hip flexor stretches. Shortened muscles can lack strength in the same way as lengthened ones, and strengthening hip flexors can be useful as part of an overall programme to strengthen the lower limb.

Making Hip Flexion More Functional

Every time you lift your leg, the hip flexors contract. The higher the leg is lifted, the greater the amount of strength is needed. Other than when climbing stairs, there are few times in everyday life when significant hip flexor strength is required. Obviously, people who play sports require greater hip flexor strength and should be referred to a professional who is able to assist with this.

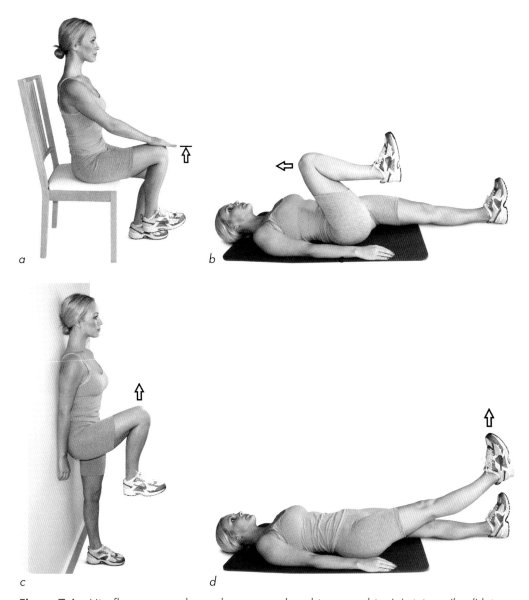

a   b   c   d

Figure 7.6 Hip flexor strength can be assessed and improved in *(a)* sitting, *(b, d)* lying and *(c)* standing positions.

Courtesy of Tim Allardyce, Rehabmypatient.com.

Water-Based Exercise

For an all-around hip strengthening programme, consider water-based exercise. Water provides resistance to movement, and pool-based exercises are valuable because they can be used in the very early stages of recovery to improve hip mobility and strength. Simply walking across the pool forwards, backwards and sideways is a great way to strengthen all of the major muscles of the hips. Lying on one's back to perform straight-leg abduction and adduction movements can be useful to strengthen the abductors and adductors, respectively.

Quick Questions

1. When using the bridge exercise to test a client's hip extensor strength, what three things might you look for to identify if there is weakness?
2. Which two functional exercises are described in the text to strengthen hip abductors?
3. What is the advantage of testing the strength of hip adductors bilaterally in the frog-like supine position?
4. Whether using the standing or supine position, which requires more strength – hip flexion with the knee flexed or hip flexion with the knee extended?
5. Why are water-based exercises helpful for someone with a hip problem?

Knees

Learning Outcomes

After reading this chapter, you should be able to do the following:

- Demonstrate simple tests to determine the strength of the knee flexor and extensor muscles.
- Show examples of knee strengthening exercises.
- Teach knee strengthening exercises in prone, supine, sitting and standing positions.
- Explain how to make any of the exercises in this chapter harder or easier.
- List examples of functional knee exercises.
- Tell which exercises in this chapter are also appropriate for the treatment of hamstring strains, tight hamstrings, hamstring cramping and tight quadriceps.
- Identify which knee strengthening exercises may also be appropriate for common conditions affecting the ankle.

This chapter focuses on exercises to strengthen the knee. These exercises are suitable for the treatment of conditions such as osteoarthritis in the knee and after knee surgery. Strengthening of the opposing muscle groups can be useful in the treatment of hamstring cramping, tight hamstrings and tight quadriceps, and although strengthening cannot affect overall knee posture, it might be helpful in improving balance for people with genu recurvatum, genu flexum, genu varum and genu valgum knee postures. Many of the exercises in this chapter are also useful in the treatment of ankle or foot problems, where strength and stability in the knee are essential to recovery or where maintaining knee function is required for everyday activities.

Testing Knee Strength

The tests described in this chapter demonstrate how to test pure movements of the knee – flexion (bending) and extension (straightening). However, as you know, we use our knees to perform everyday tasks, and these require not just strength but flexibility and balance – changing from a sitting to standing position (or sitting down from a standing position), using stairs, pressing the brake pedal when driving, squatting to put on footwear or pick something up from the ground and so on. It is important to remember this when determining a person's knee strength. The ability to perform everyday tasks can also be used as a determinant of recovery.

Knee strength may be tested by the client simply bending or straightening their knee, or it may be tested against added resistance – usually provided by the therapist or a rubber exercise band. Actively moving the knee may sound easy, but testing strength actively is very useful in the early stages of rehabilitation or after prolonged immobilisation, when there may be a significant loss of strength. Active knee flexion is a useful way to test the strength of the hamstrings after a hamstring strain, and active knee extension is a good way to test the strength of the quadriceps after a quadriceps strain, especially in the early stages of recovery.

Testing knee strength without added resistance relies on feedback from the client – the client tells you how difficult they feel a movement is and whether there is a deficit between their left and right knees. You can often observe for yourself how much effort the client appears to put into performing the movement and identify the degree of movement through which the client is able to flex or extend their knee.

Testing the strength of the knee flexors and extensors can be performed in prone, sitting, supine or standing positions, the same positions you might be using for range-of-motion exercises to increase mobility in the joint. Certain test positions are slightly more challenging than others, and these are detailed in the sections that follow. Which test position you use will depend on the client. For example, when treating a client with balance issues, you might avoid testing them in a standing position. Conversely, in later stages of recovery, you may decide to use a standing position for strength training specifically to challenge and improve the client's balance.

Knee Flexors

Identifying Weakness in the Knee Flexors

Knee flexion occurs when the heel is pulled towards the buttock. The client can bend each knee in the prone (figure 8.1) or supine (figure 8.2) positions and let you know whether they perceive a strength deficit between their left and right knees when they do this. The prone position is not suitable for clients who struggle to get into or rest in this position. Also, do not use the prone position if there is any soft tissue trauma to the front of the knee, because it may be uncomfortable for the client to rest with the knee against the treatment plinth. A client could be tested when standing, but note that in the standing position, more effort is required during knee flexion to lift the heel at the end of the movement, whereas in the prone position, more effort is required at the start of the movement. You may therefore get different results depending on your test position. For a healthy individual, this test is easy, but after an injury, it may be difficult and you may wish to begin with a client seated, for example.

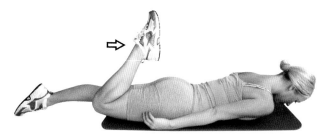

Figure 8.1 Active knee flexion in the prone position.
Courtesy of Tim Allardyce, Rehabmypatient.com.

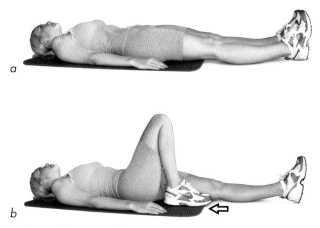

Figure 8.2 Active knee flexion in the supine position.
Courtesy of Tim Allardyce, Rehabmypatient.com.

TIP

If there appears to be a deficit in a client's ability to perform knee flexion actively, it is important to determine whether this is due to lack of strength or to restriction of the joint.

Oedema can restrict flexion, as is common after injury or surgery to the knee, but flexion can also be restricted in healthy individuals who have extremely large muscles; where the hamstrings and calf muscles are well developed, when brought together in knee flexion, they may prevent the knee from fully flexing. However, you would expect an equal restriction on both the left and right knees if the restriction were due to bulky muscles. This would also be the case when assessing someone with a high body mass index, where fat deposits around the knee may restrict flexion on both knees.

The prone and supine positions are the easiest positions in which to apply manual resistance to the muscles and thus compare strength between the left and right muscle groups. To do this, simply stand at the foot end of the plinth and cup your hand around the client's ankle. Then, ask your client to try to bend their knee or 'bring the heel to the buttock' whilst you apply the resistance. As a therapist, you have strong leverage in these positions, which are therefore good positions in which to test the knee flexors of a client in whom you suspect these muscles are strong (a rugby player, for example).

Knee Flexor Strengthening

Strengthening of the knee flexors is important for people with osteoarthritis in the knee and after surgery to the knee. It is also important for the recovery from a hamstring strain. Knee flexors can be strengthened by adding resistance in the sitting (figure 8.3a) or prone (figure 8.3b) positions using a rubber exercise band. Begin with a straight knee, and slowly bend the knee against the resistance. Bending the knee against gravity (figure 8.4) is slightly more functional and may not require added resistance. Many clients benefit from holding a tabletop or chair back for balance.

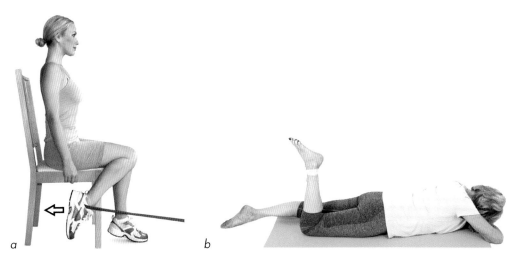

a   b

Figure 8.3 Strengthening the knee flexors using a rubber exercise band in the (a) sitting or (b) prone position.

Courtesy of Tim Allardyce, Rehabmypatient.com.

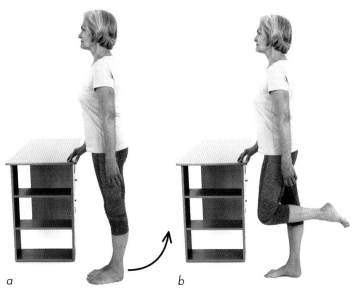

Figure 8.4 Strengthening the knee flexors in a standing position.

Courtesy of Tim Allardyce, Rehabmypatient.com.

TIP

The hamstrings tend to cramp when shortened. A quick way to overcome this is to contract the quadriceps or the hip flexors, using the knee extension exercises shown in the next section.

Knee Extensors

Identifying Weakness in the Knee Extensors

Knee extension occurs when the leg is straightened. One of the simplest tests of knee extension strength is the degree to which a client can straighten their leg when seated (figure 8.5). This requires no added resistance but can require effort because the leg is being lifted against gravity.

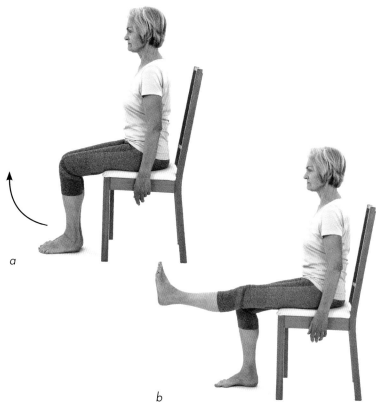

a

b

Figure 8.5 Testing knee extension in the sitting position.

Courtesy of Tim Allardyce, Rehabmypatient.com.

An easy way to test knee extension strength by adding manual resistance is to start with your client in the prone position and with their knee flexed (figure 8.1); place your hand on the anterior of the ankle and ask the client to try to straighten the knee, bringing their ankle back down to the treatment couch.

TIP

In the early stages of recovery, it is rarely necessary to apply any resistance to the ankle when using the exercise shown in figure 8.5. However, in later recovery stages, you could add resistance by simply placing your hand on the anterior of the client's ankle before they begin to straighten the knee.

Knee Extensor Strengthening

Knee extension exercises are important for regaining general knee strength but are also useful for overcoming cramping in the hamstrings. This is because the quadriceps (along with the hip flexors) are the antagonists to the hamstrings, and contraction of the anterior thigh muscles reduces tone in the posterior thigh. These exercises are important for people with osteoarthritis in the knee and after knee surgery. All of the weight-bearing exercises illustrated in this section are also suitable as part of an ankle strengthening programme – provided, of course, that there are no contraindications (such as an unhealed fracture).

When your goal is strengthening the knee extensors, a useful exercise to begin with is performed in the supine position with a small towel rolled up beneath the knee. The aim of the exercise is to straighten the leg (figure 8.6). This requires the knee extensors to work in a small range of movement. The value of this exercise is that it can be performed when a person cannot sit or stand, perhaps due to weakness in the knee extensors, and it is therefore especially helpful in the early stages of recovery from injury. With or without the towel, this exercise is also helpful when trying to overcome genu flexum, sometimes caused by contraction of the soft tissues at the back of the knee. Compare this to figure 8.5. Notice how, in that figure, the knee is moved through a greater range.

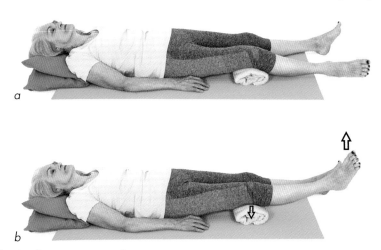

Figure 8.6 Performing supine knee extension.
Courtesy of Tim Allardyce, Rehabmypatient.com.

If your client is able to flex their hip to approximately 90 degrees, they could practise knee extension in that position (figure 8.5). This requires lifting the foot through 90 degrees against gravity and can be a good way to progress knee extension exercises when a client is unable to bear weight. With the hip flexed and the knee extended, this exercise has the added advantage of helping to assist with lymphatic drainage, and this could help reduce swelling in the knee. The exercise does, however, require good hamstring flexibility.

If your client is able, resting in the prone position can also be used. In this position, the knee is straightened against the resistance of a rubber exercise band (figure 8.7). This requires your client to be able to hold an exercise band in one hand.

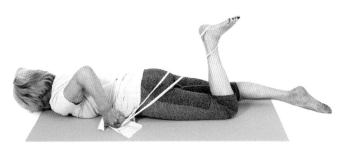

Figure 8.7   Knee extension against resistance in the prone position.

Courtesy of Tim Allardyce, Rehabmypatient.com.

Functional Knee Exercises

One of the exercises commonly overlooked is that of simply trying to stand, with or without support. In standing, knee extensor strength is required simply to keep the leg straight, and this can be very difficult after injury. This is a useful exercise if a person does not yet have the strength or balance to walk far from a chair or bed. Also, because this exercise requires weight bearing through both legs, the client can gradually increase the amount of weight they place through the affected knee. Using the hands to press up from a seated position is a good approach to start with, but eventually, the client should be encouraged to stand without the aid of their arms. One way to encourage this is to place the arms across the chest (figure 8.8).

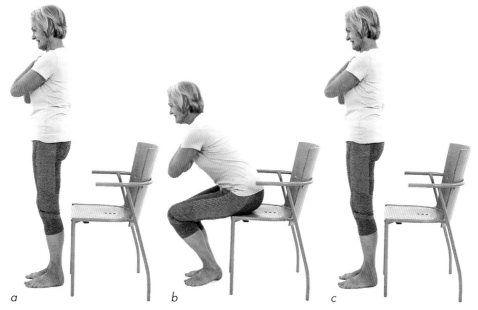

a   b   c

Figure 8.8   Practising the sit-to-stand exercise.

Courtesy of Tim Allardyce, Rehabmypatient.com.

TIP

Sitting down from a standing position requires more effort than standing from a seated position. This is because the quadriceps are required to work eccentrically as we lower our body to a seat, and this is challenging. Therefore, one way to progress this exercise is to stand quickly, then slowly lower down. A different way to progress the exercise is to place more weight through the affected knee, rather than keeping the weight evenly distributed. This has the effect of helping to strengthen that knee whilst performing an exercise that is relatively stable. Even more challenging is a single-leg sit-to-stand movement.

Once a client is able to stand, they could progress to performing small squats using a wall for support (figure 8.9). For some people, this is more challenging than the simple sit-to-stand exercise because it requires balance. The value of squatting in this manner is that weight is distributed between both legs, making the exercise easier and more stable than one-leg movements.

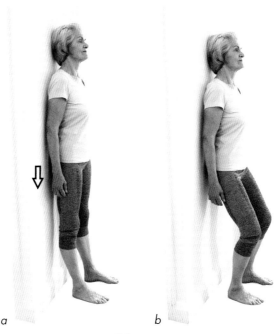

a   b

Figure 8.9 Miniature squats using a wall for support.

Courtesy of Tim Allardyce, Rehabmypatient.com.

TIP

A way to progress the squatting exercise is to perform miniature squats without a wall, deeper squats using a wall, and then deeper squats without a wall.

Once someone can perform miniature squats, they could also progress to a split squat, with the affected knee foremost. Using a chair back or tabletop for support, the client should place one leg in front of the other and then perform the squat (figure 8.10), lowering the body only a little. Once the client can perform a small split squat, they could progress by lowering more and deepening the lunge (figure 8.11). These small lunges are a preferable starting point compared to full lunges, which require considerable strength and balance.

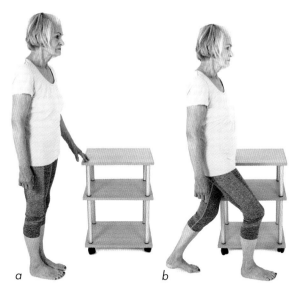

Figure 8.10 Performing a miniature split squat.
Courtesy of Tim Allardyce, Rehabmypatient.com.

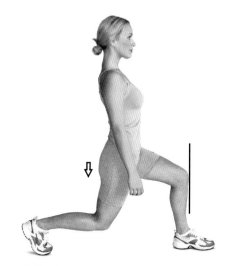

Figure 8.11 Performing a full split squat.
Courtesy of Tim Allardyce, Rehabmypatient.com.

TIP

In the lunge position, it is important that the knee remains over the ankle and does not advance farther forwards than the position of the ankle (figure 8.11). A way to encourage this is to have the client drop the back knee towards the ground rather than lunging forwards.

Walking is a simple way to improve balance and strength in the knee. The value of walking with an aid, such as a stick, should not be underestimated; an aid can provide stability, which can increase the duration a person can walk. Many people are reluctant to use walking aids, perhaps due to their association with aging. If you are working with a client who does not want to use an aid outdoors, perhaps encourage them to use it indoors at least. This could make the difference between the client remaining predominantly sedentary or using the aid to move around within their home.

Practising small, single-leg bends is another functional exercise (figure 8.12). For some clients, this may be too challenging because all of the weight is placed through the knee. However, in later stages of rehabilitation, this may be exactly what is required. Performing this exercise more slowly makes it more difficult. To progress this further, the client could flex the knee to a greater degree.

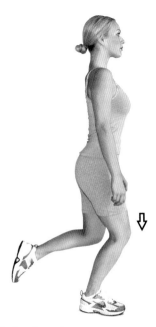

Figure 8.12 Practising a single-leg bend.
Courtesy of Tim Allardyce, Rehabmypatient.com.

An obvious functional exercise is stepping up or stair climbing. In the early stages of recovery, it is helpful to have a handrail (figure 8.13). This is a challenging exercise because it requires lifting the entire body up against gravity using one knee at a time. Therefore, to make the exercise easier, use steps that are small in height, and to make it more difficult, use a higher step.

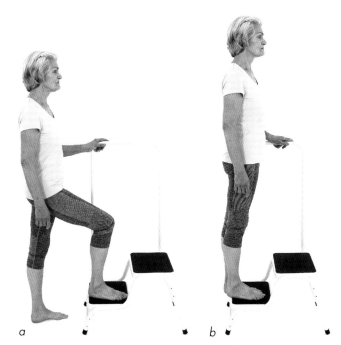

Figure 8.13 Stepping up with support.

Courtesy of Tim Allardyce, Rehabmypatient.com.

TIP

Stepping down is much harder than stepping up. This is because the extensors of the supporting knee are required to work eccentrically when stepping down. Therefore, if your aim is to make the exercise more difficult, encourage the client to step down slowly, controlling the movement with the affected leg.

Water-Based Exercises

Knee strengthening can be performed in water by practising flexion and extension or 'cycling' types of movements. Exercise in water has the advantage of being non–weight-bearing and therefore forms a valuable component of early rehabilitation. Exercising in water can help make some of the movements accessible for people who would not be able to perform them on land. Double-leg and single-leg squats can be performed more easily in water than on land, for example.

Balance Exercises

Please refer to chapter 9 for balance exercises. Balance is commonly affected after an injury to the knee and in people with conditions such as knee osteoarthritis. Balance exercises are an important part of knee rehabilitation and can help maintain or improve a person's existing ability to balance.

Quick Questions

1. Other than weakness in the knee flexor muscles, what are three things that might restrict knee flexion when it is tested actively?
2. When testing the strength of the knee extensors in either the sitting or prone position, to which part of the lower limb would you apply gentle pressure to add resistance?
3. What is one advantage and one disadvantage of performing an exercise to strengthen the knee extensors in the supine position with the hip flexed to approximately 90 degrees?
4. Why is the stand-to-sit exercise harder to perform than the sit-to-stand exercise?
5. Name three ways you could progress someone who is now able to perform a miniature squat against a wall, still using a squat-type exercise.

Feet and Ankles

Learning Outcomes

After reading this chapter, you should be able to do the following:

- Demonstrate simple tests to determine the strength of the ankle flexor, extensor, evertor and invertor muscles.
- Teach simple exercises to strengthen the ankle flexors, extensors, evertors and invertors.
- Explain how to make any of the exercises in this chapter harder or easier.
- Illustrate a safe, simple way to test balance.
- Select and demonstrate exercises that are appropriate for common conditions affecting the ankle.
- Demonstrate ankle strengthening exercises in supine, sitting and standing positions.
- List examples of functional ankle strengthening exercises.
- Tell which exercises in this chapter are also appropriate for the treatment of common leg conditions: calf muscle strain, tight calf muscles, calf cramping, shin splints, and tight tibialis anterior and peroneal (fibular) muscles.

The muscles of the ankle bring about different movements: plantar flexion, dorsiflexion, eversion and inversion. The plantar flexors are much stronger than the other muscles of the ankle because they need to be able to lift the entire body when pushing off during walking or raising up onto the toes. The dorsiflexors, by contrast, only have to raise the toes up a little to prevent their catching on the ground during walking, and even less strength is required in the evertors and invertors. However, a common mistake is to focus on strengthening only the plantar flexors, when it is in fact important to strengthen all the muscles of the ankle. Together, these muscles provide stability to the joint and are important for balance.

Weakness in all the ankle muscles is common after periods of immobilisation – for example, when someone has sustained a lower limb injury or has been ill. The longer a person has been unable to use their ankle, the greater the degree of muscle weakness

225

and the longer it will take to improve this. The exercises provided in this chapter are useful for the treatment of the conditions described in chapter 6, predominantly ankle sprains, Achilles tendinopathy, ankle fractures, stiff ankles, plantar fasciitis and stiff feet. Chapter 6 also covered the postural conditions known as pes planus, pes cavus, pes valgus and pes varus, and a few of the exercises in this chapter are relevant for those conditions also.

Strengthening of the ankle muscles is important in the treatment of many conditions, not only after an injury or immobilisation. For example, a quick way to overcome cramping in the calf is to contract the antagonist muscle group – the dorsiflexors. Therefore, you will find the section on how to strengthen ankle dorsiflexors useful if you are treating people prone to calf cramping. The exercises presented in this chapter are likely to be helpful in the treatment of the conditions described in chapter 5 – calf muscle strain, tight calf muscles, calf cramping, shin splints and tight tibialis anterior and peroneal (fibular) muscles.

Testing Ankle Strength

The easiest way to test ankle strength is to ask your client to perform one of the ranges of movement – plantar flexion, dorsiflexion, eversion or inversion – against resistance. Resistance could be in the form of the client's own body weight, a resistance band, a wall or even resistance provided by you. The form of resistance you use depends on factors such as the degree of weakness you suspect and the client's overall state of health.

For example, to test the strength of the plantar flexors of someone recovering from a severe ankle sprain, you might ask them to perform a toe raise whilst they are sitting and let you know whether their ankle feels weak. You might also ask them to lie face down or supine on a treatment plinth and to plantar flex as you apply resistance to the foot whilst you assess for any strength deficits. You should not ask them to attempt to perform a single-leg calf raise, because they will almost certainly lack the strength to do this, which could be demotivating. They are also likely to lack balance.

The strengthening exercises in this chapter are presented in order from easiest to hardest as much as possible. Therefore, to test a person's strength, you could select the very first exercise initially but would be unlikely to select the last. However, the degree of difficulty in performing an exercise will depend on the condition you are treating and the general health of the client. For example, a bilateral toe raise with straight legs may be easier than a bilateral toe raise with bent knees if someone is recovering from a torn soleus muscle, because the bent-knee position requires the soleus muscle to work harder to bring about plantar flexion than does the straight-leg position.

Plantar Flexors

Plantar Flexor Muscle Strengthening

One of the easiest ways to strengthen the plantar flexors is to lift the heels off the ground whilst seated (figure 9.1). This is the kind of exercise that might be appropriate after a prolonged period of immobilisation, when the ankle will be especially weak and the person is likely to have very poor balance. Because this exercise involves lifting only the weight of the lower legs and partial weight of the thighs, the advantages are that it is manageable for most people, does not need to be performed bilaterally and does not require balance. Therefore, it is generally a safe exercise to use and a good one with which to start.

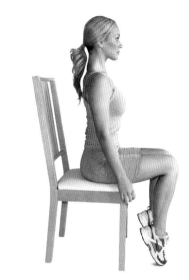

Figure 9.1 Strengthening the plantar flexors using minimal resistance.

Courtesy of Tim Allardyce, Rehabmypatient.com.

TIP

To progress this exercise, the client could simply place their hands on their knees whilst leaning forwards slightly, thus using their own body weight to apply some resistance.

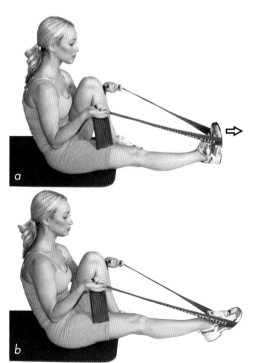

Another way to strengthen the plantar flexors is using a resistance band. In this exercise, the client begins with their foot in dorsiflexion (figure 9.2a) and then plantar flexes against the resistance of the band (figure 9.2b). This exercise can be performed sitting on the floor or on a chair.

Using body weight as the resistance is an effective way to strengthen the plantar flexors, but it can be challenging. A good way for the client to start is by holding on to a chair for balance and rising up onto the toes bilaterally (figure 9.3a). Note that the exercise may feel different if the feet are turned in (figure 9.3b) or out (figure 9.3c).

Figure 9.2 Using a resistance band to strengthen the plantar flexors: (a) Begin in dorsiflexion and (b) gently plantar flex.

Courtesy of Tim Allardyce, Rehabmypatient.com.

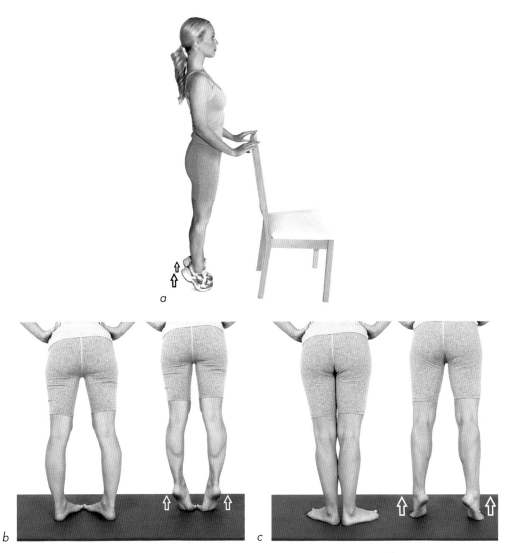

Figure 9.3 Strengthening the plantar flexors when standing with the feet in a *(a)* neutral, *(b)* toe-in or *(c)* toe-out position.

Courtesy of Tim Allardyce, Rehabmypatient.com.

TIP

A single-leg raise should be used only when a person can comfortably perform a bilateral toe raise with no pain.

It is interesting to compare a straight-leg toe raise with a bent-knee toe raise. In the bent-knee position (figure 9.4), the soleus must work harder than in the straight-leg position. This exercise could be useful when working with people recovering from a soleus strain. It can also be useful to help determine if there is any strength deficit in the soleus.

Eccentric calf training is a commonly used exercise for ankle rehabilitation. It requires a step or stair, preferably with a handrail for balance. It can be performed with a small towel beneath the toes (see figure 9.5) or without. In this exercise, the client begins on tiptoe (figure 9.5a) and slowly lowers their heels to beneath the level of the step (figure 9.5b). This movement requires eccentric contraction of the calf and is more challenging than plantar flexion (which involves concentric contraction).

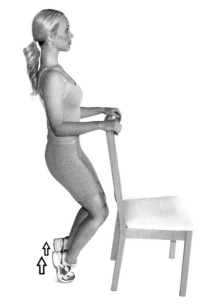

Figure 9.4 Strengthening the soleus.
Courtesy of Tim Allardyce, Rehabmypatient.com.

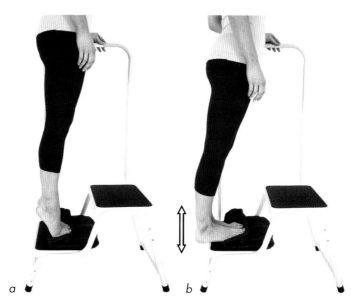

Figure 9.5 Performing an eccentric calf contraction exercise (a) begins on tiptoe and (b) ends in dorsiflexion.
Courtesy of Tim Allardyce, Rehabmypatient.com.

Dorsiflexors

Dorsiflexor Muscle Strengthening

In either a sitting (figure 9.6) or lying position, a simple way to strengthen the ankle dorsiflexors is for the client to apply resistance to the ankle using their other foot as they attempt to dorsiflex. If this proves difficult, a resistance band can be used. This exercise often works best in the supine position (figure 9.7) with the band wrapped around a secure anchor or being held by someone else. Activation of the ankle dorsiflexors is a quick way to overcome cramping in the calf. If a client can bear weight through the ankle, then walking on the heels (figure 9.8) is another possibility.

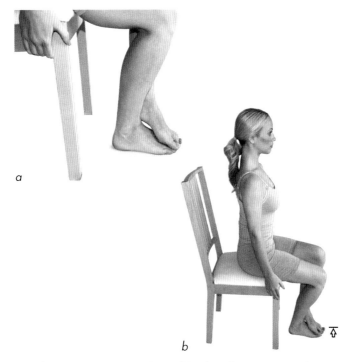

a

b

Figure 9.6 *(a)* Applying resistance to the ankle dorsiflexors using the opposite foot whilst *(b)* trying to raise the bottom foot.

Courtesy of Tim Allardyce, Rehabmypatient.com.

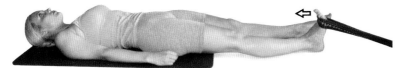

Figure 9.7   Using a resistance band to strengthen the ankle dorsiflexors.
Courtesy of Tim Allardyce, Rehabmypatient.com.

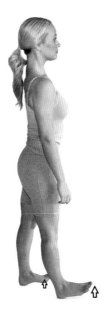

Figure 9.8   Heel walking to strengthen the dorsiflexors.
Courtesy of Tim Allardyce, Rehabmypatient.com.

Evertors

Evertor Muscle Strengthening

Most people find eversion of the ankle more difficult than plantar flexion or dorsiflexion, perhaps because eversion is a relatively small movement. Strengthening the evertors is crucial after a lateral ankle sprain. In a systematic review, Wagemans and colleagues (2022) concluded that exercise rehabilitation reduces the risk of reinjury after a lateral ankle sprain but that there was insufficient evidence to determine the optimal content of a rehabilitation programme. Although unilateral exercises could be used to strengthen the evertors, bilateral exercises are preferable because they are simply much easier to perform, irrespective of the amount of existing ankle strength. For example, when lying or sitting (figure 9.9a), the client can cross the feet at the ankles and use the feet to oppose eversion or can use a resistance band looped around the ankles (figure 9.9b) to provide the resistance.

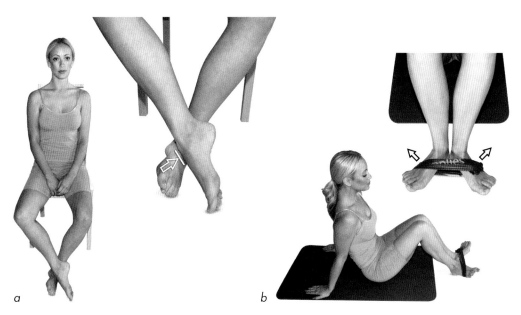

a   b

Figure 9.9 Exercises to strengthen the ankle evertors using (a) self-resistance or (b) a resistance band.

Courtesy of Tim Allardyce, Rehabmypatient.com.

Invertors

Invertor Muscle Strengthening

Similarly to eversion, inversion is a movement many people find difficult to perform compared to plantar flexion or dorsiflexion because the ankle has less movement into inversion than into plantar flexion or dorsiflexion. The invertors are important muscles and contribute to balance; therefore, there is a good rationale for strengthening them. An easy way to strengthen the invertors is by using a resistance band. The band is placed around the foot, and the client inverts the ankle against the resistance (figure 9.10). This exercise could be performed sitting on the floor, as shown in figure 9.10, or in a chair or bed.

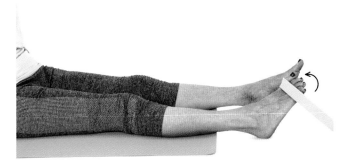

Figure 9.10   Using a resistance band to strengthen the ankle invertor muscles.
Courtesy of Tim Allardyce, Rehabmypatient.com.

Balance Exercises

When someone stops using their lower limbs, whether this is due to illness or to an injury affecting the hip, thigh, knee, ankle or foot, the muscles start to deteriorate, and the person loses not only strength but balance. Poor balance increases the risk of injury, and this is especially significant for older adults or those with osteoporosis, in whom the risk of fracture from falls is significant. Fortunately, many exercises can be used to improve balance, and the simplest and most effective of these are shown in the following sections.

Testing Balance

The single-leg standing exercise (figure 9.11) can be used to both test and improve balance.

Balance is impaired not only after an injury to the ankle but also when there are issues affecting the knee or even the hip. Therefore, the material in this section will also be useful when helping people to recover from hip and knee conditions.

To test or improve balance, ask your client to stand with their feet hip distance apart. Next, ask them to shift their weight onto the non-affected lower limb, then to flex the knee of that leg slightly. Once the knee is slightly flexed, ask them to lift their other foot off the floor, transferring all their weight onto the non-affected side. They do not need to lift the affected limb high off the floor, but they should prevent it from touching the leg on which they are balancing (see figure 9.11). Note the amount of time they can remain in this position. You may wish to try this three times and determine the average duration. It can be helpful to ask your client to keep a diary, noting improvements in the length of time they can perform the one-leg balance exercise. This exercise strengthens leg muscles, and it is normal for the client to experience some aching in the leg in the following 2 days, as with all strength training.

Because we use our eyes to help us balance, practising the single-leg standing exercise with the eyes closed creates more of a challenge. To make balance exercises safer when the eyes are closed, it is helpful to perform them where there is a handhold nearby – a table surface or the back of a chair, for example. You need to determine for yourself whether practising with the eyes closed will be safe for your client.

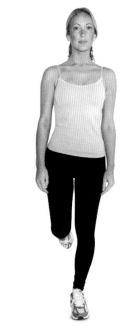

Figure 9.11 The single-leg stand to test and improve balance.

Courtesy of Tim Allardyce, Rehabmypatient.com.

After the client performs the one-leg balance exercise on the non-affected side, have them repeat it on the affected side. There are two ways to determine whether balance is impaired in this position. In most cases, either your client will not be able to balance on the affected side (or the length of time they can stand on that leg will be significantly reduced) or they may be able to balance but with a lot of wobbling and use of the arms to maintain the position. The simplest way to improve balance is to practise this exercise.

There are many ways that this exercise can be progressed. A common mistake is to progress too quickly, such as by using a 'wobble' board – an unstable board that wobbles when a person stands on it, thus challenging balance. However, if used too soon, this increases the risk of reinjury. There are many other, safer ways to challenge balance and improve strength in the ankle at the same time.

One of the best ways to progress the single-leg standing exercise is to have the client practise it whilst standing on a sloped surface rather than flat ground. When we face uphill or downhill or stand with our side towards the top or bottom of a hill, force passes through different parts of the ankle. An easy way to progress the balance exercise is simply to have the client practise it when standing on a gentle slope, facing different directions.

Another way to challenge balance is to stand on an uneven surface or a surface with a different texture. For example, standing on a wooden floor provides more support than standing on a thick carpet or on a rolled-up towel.

Items such as a wobble board should only be used once a person can balance on different static slopes and surfaces.

It is important to challenge balance safely. One exercise you may wish to try is the clock exercise. Have your client imagine they are standing in the centre of a clock that is drawn on the ground (figure 9.12). When standing on the affected limb, have them use the toes of the non-affected limb to point to where various numbers would be on the clock. This requires movement of the non-affected limb away from the midline, making it more challenging to maintain balance.

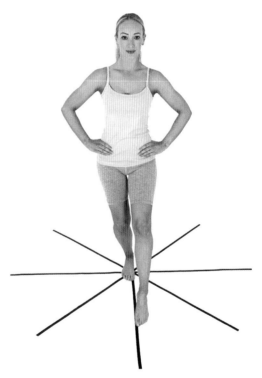

Figure 9.12 The 'clock' exercise to challenge balance.

Courtesy of Tim Allardyce, Rehabmypatient.com.

Functional Exercises to Strengthen the Ankle and Improve Balance

Exercises that are more representative of everyday use of the ankle are those that combine both strength and balance, such as standing on one leg whilst brushing one's teeth or hair. For some people, this may be too challenging. An easier exercise might be to simply stand with one leg in front of the other and sway forwards and backwards, placing weight first on the front leg and then on the back leg (figure 9.13). It is important to alternate the leg that is in front, but it does not matter whether the affected or non-affected leg is positioned in front to begin. This could be progressed to walking in a straight line as if on a tightrope (figure 9.14).

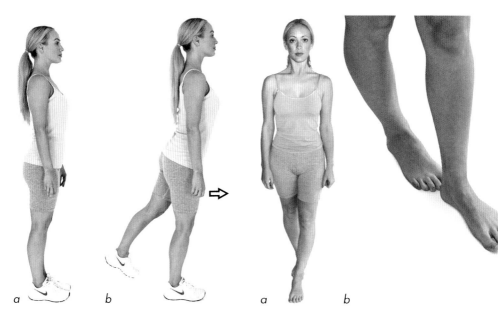

Figure 9.13 Weight transfer forwards and backwards.

Courtesy of Tim Allardyce, Rehabmypatient.com.

Figure 9.14 Walking as if on a tightrope to challenge balance.

Courtesy of Tim Allardyce, Rehabmypatient.com.

FUNCTIONAL ANKLE EXERCISES

Positioning the legs hip distance apart and transferring weight from side to side (figure 9.15) is another way to make strengthening exercises more functional.

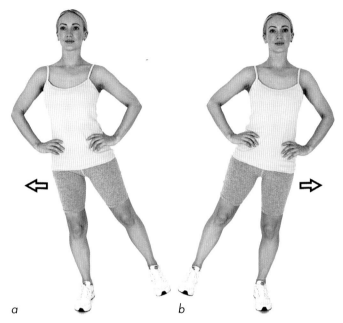

a   b

Figure 9.15   Weight transfer side to side.

Courtesy of Tim Allardyce, Rehabmypatient.com.

Finally, all kinds of exercises can be used to improve strength and balance simply by introducing movement in different positions, such as leaning forwards on one leg.

Exercises to Strengthen the Feet and Toes

It is difficult to separate exercises for the feet and toes from those of the ankle, because the toes contain not only small, intrinsic muscles but also muscles that attach to the leg via the ankle: the long toe flexors and extensors and the evertors and invertors of the ankle. Therefore, many of the preceding exercises will also help to strengthen the feet and toes, and certain exercises may be helpful to strengthen the flexors of the toes specifically. Whilst the exercises in this chapter may have little effect, if any, on pes varus, pes valgus and pes cavus foot postures, the exercises that follow may be helpful for people with pes planus (flatfoot).

One way to treat pes planus caused by faulty postural activity of the foot muscles is to stand barefoot, with the feet hip distance apart, then consciously contract the buttock muscles. Notice how contraction of the buttocks lifts the medial arches of the feet.

To strengthen the tibialis posterior and the long toe flexors, toe flexion could be performed against the resistance of an exercise band. One way to do this is to dorsiflex the ankle, then place the flat band along the length of the foot (figure 9.16a). Whilst holding the band taut, flex the toes against it (figure 9.16b).

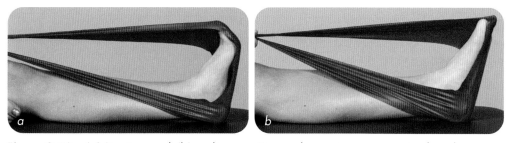

Figure 9.16 *(a)* Starting and *(b)* ending positions when using an exercise band to strengthen the long toe flexors.

Some clients find it fun to try foot gymnastics, which are commonly prescribed for flexible pes planus despite little evidence that they are effective. Examples of exercises used in foot gymnastics are using the feet and toes to tie a knot in a rope, using the toes to pick up and fasten a clothes peg to a line or to the edge of a cup, passing a stick or pencil back and forth with a partner, holding a paper cup between the toes of one foot whilst using the toes of the other foot to pick up small objects and deposit these in the cup or using the toes to pick up small hoops and place them over a pole. A simple way to begin might be to try picking up a facecloth or a small towel (figure 9.17).

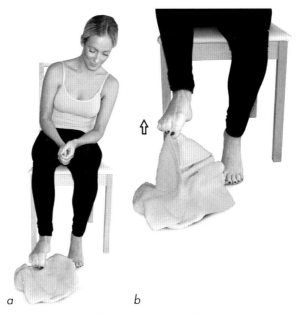

a   b

Figure 9.17 Using the toes to pick up a small towel to strengthen the toe flexors.
Courtesy of Tim Allardyce, Rehabmypatient.com.

Quick Questions

1. List three advantages of a seated calf raise when treating someone with weak ankles or poor balance.
2. Which ankle muscles does heel walking strengthen?
3. Why might it be preferable to perform ankle evertor exercises bilaterally?
4. When the single-leg standing test is used, what two things indicate that someone has poor balance?
5. Give examples of foot strengthening exercises used in foot gymnastics.

Lower Limb Postural Assessment Chart

Use this lower limb postural assessment chart to document your observations, recording these in the appropriate column depending on whether what you observe affects the right or the left side of the body.

ANTERIOR VIEW		
Right side	**Posture**	**Left side**
	Stance	
	Lateral tilt of the pelvis	

ANTERIOR VIEW

Right side	Posture	Left side

Pelvic rotation

Muscle bulk and tone

Genu varum or genu valgum?

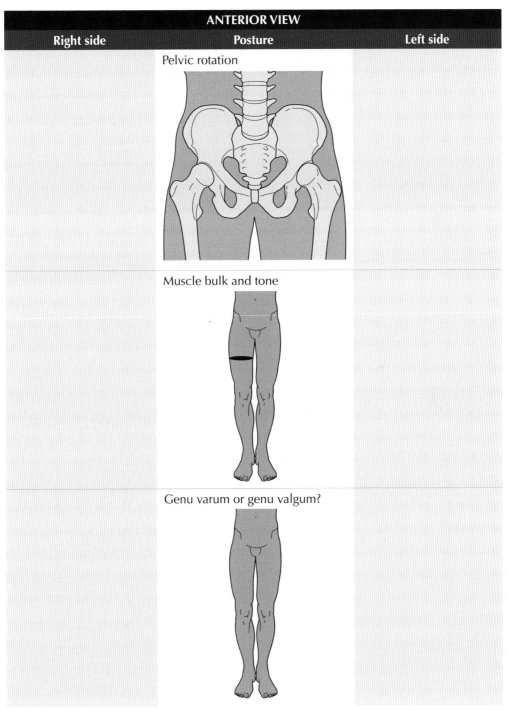

(continued)

Lower Limb Postural Assessment Chart *(continued)*

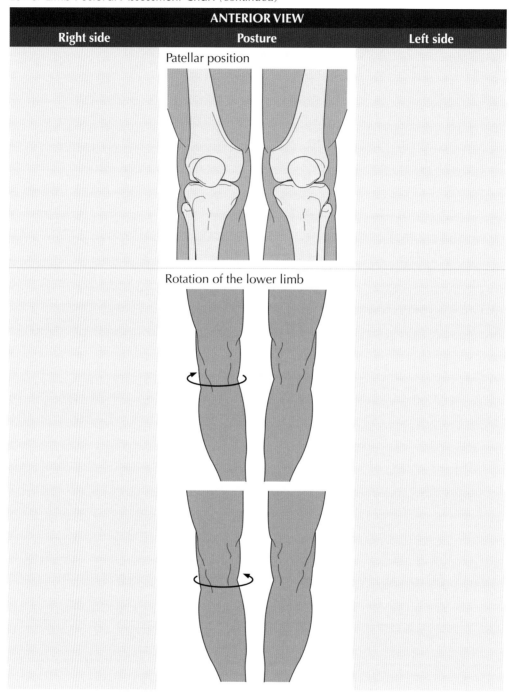

	ANTERIOR VIEW	
Right side	Posture	Left side
	Patellar position	
	Rotation of the lower limb	

ANTERIOR VIEW		
Right side	Posture	Left side

Tibial torsion

Q angle

- Anterior superior iliac spine
- Q angle
- Midpoint of the patella
- Tibial tuberosity

Ankles

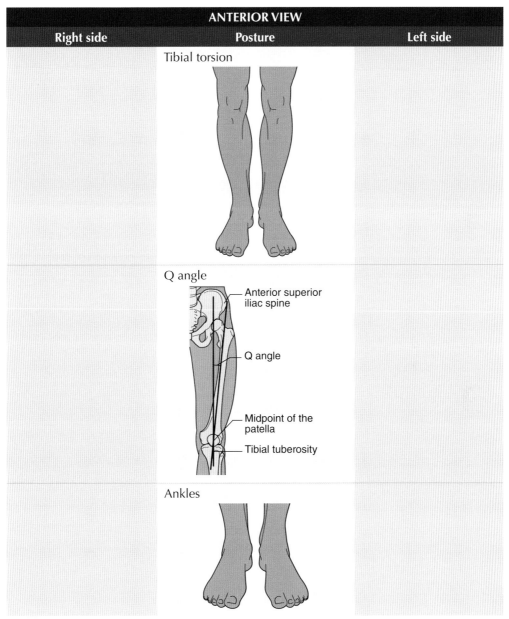

(continued)

Lower Limb Postural Assessment Chart *(continued)*

ANTERIOR VIEW		
Right side	**Posture**	**Left side**
	Foot position 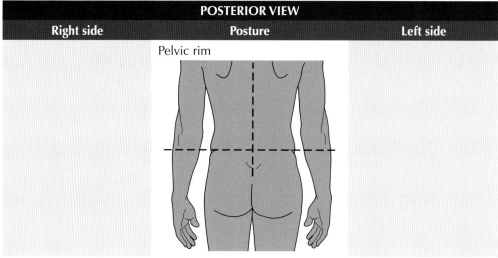	
	Other observations	

POSTERIOR VIEW		
Right side	**Posture**	**Left side**
	Pelvic rim	

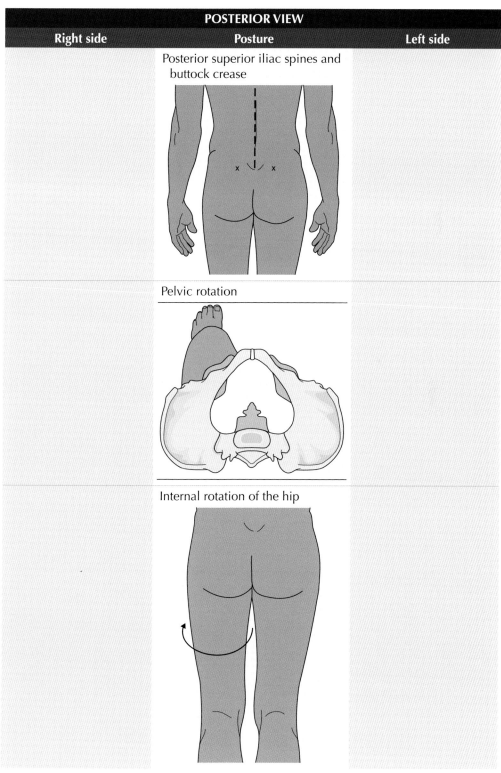

Lower Limb Postural Assessment Chart *(continued)*

POSTERIOR VIEW		
Right side	**Posture**	**Left side**
	Muscle bulk and tone	
	Posterior knee	
	Calf midline	

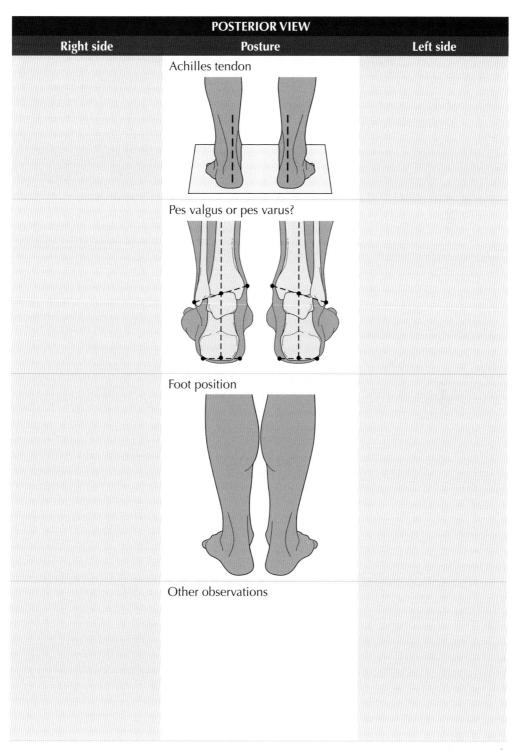

POSTERIOR VIEW		
Right side	**Posture**	**Left side**
	Achilles tendon	
	Pes valgus or pes varus?	
	Foot position	
	Other observations	

(continued)

Lower Limb Postural Assessment Chart *(continued)*

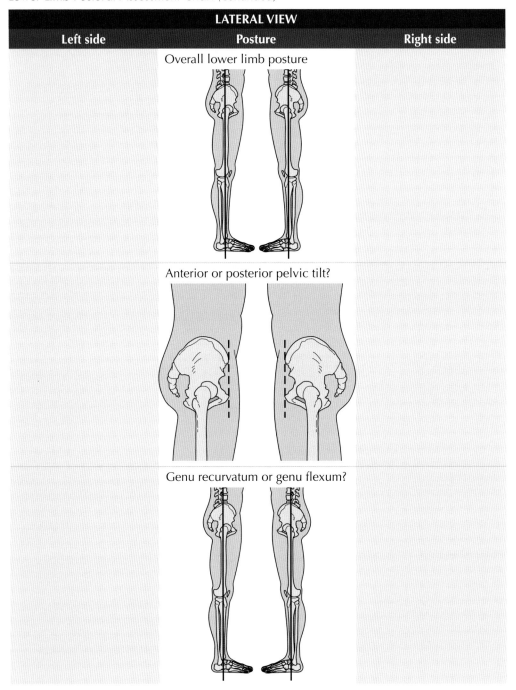

LATERAL VIEW		
Left side	**Posture**	**Right side**
	Ankles 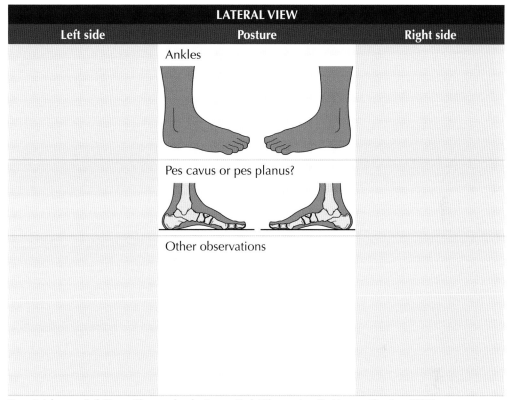	
	Pes cavus or pes planus?	
	Other observations	

From J. Johnson, *Soft Tissue Therapy for the Lower Limb* (Champaign, IL: Human Kinetics, 2025).

Chapter 1 Answers

1. When using the anterior view, it is useful to use the anterior superior iliac spines (ASIS) when assessing someone for pelvic rotation.
2. It is more accurate to measure the Q angle with a client standing rather than supine because when the client is standing, the patella is under the usual weight-bearing stresses.
3. When someone has a pelvis that is laterally tilted upwards on the right, the right hip is adducted and the left hip is abducted.
4. In the posterior view, the purpose of imagining or drawing a line down the midline of the calf is to help determine whether there is rotation in the lower limb, particularly the hip.
5. Key observations that might indicate someone has genu recurvatum posture (knee hyperextension) are a large portion of the calf falling posterior to a plumb line (in the side view), the popliteal space appearing prominent (in the posterior view) and the patella appearing to be compressed and pointing downwards (in the anterior view).

Chapter 2 Answers

1. A treatment aim is a general, overarching target, whereas a treatment goal is a specific set of steps needed to reach that target.
2. Treatment aims listed in this chapter are the following:

   Reduce pain

   Reduce swelling

   Improve balance

   Overcome the sensation of muscle stiffness

   Overcome or prevent muscle cramping

   Regain normal movement in a joint

   Improve weight bearing through the lower limb

   Improve lower limb strength

   Regain everyday lower limb function

   Educate the client

   Help correct postural imbalance
3. The pain measurement tools described in this chapter are the Visual Analogue Scale (VAS) and the Numerical Pain Rating Scale (NPRS).

4. Common lower limb muscle length tests are the prone knee bend test, straight-leg raise test, Thomas test and Ober test.

5. The Lower Extremity Functional Scale is a measure of lower limb function. The user is asked to score the level of difficulty they have, or would have, if attempting certain activities, irrespective of what lower limb condition they have.

Chapter 3 Answers

1. The sciatic nerve is affected in piriformis syndrome.

2. In a groin strain, the adductor muscles may be damaged by impact, sudden contraction or overstretching.

3. When applying a gentle passive stretch in the supine position to someone with tight left hip adductors, it is helpful for the clinician to stabilise the pelvis by placing their right hand over the client's right anterior superior iliac spine.

4. When treating someone with tight hip flexors, soft tissue release can be applied to the iliacus with the client in the side-lying position.

5. To identify the tensor fasciae latae with a client in the supine position, ask the client to lift their leg off the treatment couch and rotate the hip internally as you palpate the muscle close to the posterior side of the iliac crest.

Chapter 4 Answers

1. Signs that may identify a hamstring strain include the following:

    Pain on palpation

    Pain on stretching of the muscle

    Pain on resisted knee flexion

    Pain on resisted hip extension

    Bruising (severe cases)

    Loss of strength in knee flexion or hip extension (severe cases)

2. When a client uses soft tissue release in the supine position, dorsiflexing the ankle increases the stretch compared to when the ankle is plantar flexed.

3. When using a ball to deactivate trigger points in the sitting position, the ball should be moved after about 30 seconds.

4. When stretching the quadriceps in the prone position, placing a towel beneath the knee extends the hip and therefore enhances the stretch to one of the quadriceps muscles – the rectus femoris.

5. For some people, a foam roller is helpful for reducing sensations of quadriceps tightness.

Chapter 5 Answers

1. Actively contracting the tibialis anterior helps reduce the sensation of cramping in the calf.

2. A more accurate term for *shin splints* is *medial tibial stress syndrome*.

3. When preparing to work on trigger points in the peroneal (fibular) muscles, it is important to be aware of the peroneal nerve in the region of the head of the fibula.

4. When working with someone with osteoarthritis in the knee, soft tissue techniques should be used in conjunction with therapeutic exercise because there is not enough evidence to support the use of soft tissue techniques alone.

5. When applying tape for the treatment of genu recurvatum, the tape is applied with the knee in a neutral knee posture.

Chapter 6 Answers

1. It is necessary to educate a client with regards to the importance of rehabilitation after an ankle sprain because there is strong evidence that having had an ankle sprain is a risk factor for subsequent re-sprain.

2. When working with someone who had their ankle immobilised after a fracture, it is necessary to mobilise and stretch the joints of the foot and toes.

3. It useful to stretch the ankle joint to more than 90 degrees as part of treatment for a stiff ankle because the ankle joint needs to dorsiflex to more than 90 degrees during normal walking.

4. In the pes valgus foot posture, there is compression of the soft tissues on the lateral side of the ankle.

5. Massage is helpful when applied to the medial side of the leg, ankle and foot when working with someone with the pes varus foot posture.

Chapter 7 Answers

1. When using the bridge exercise to test a client's hip extensor strength, three things that indicate weakness are (1) the exercise appearing difficult for the person, (2) inability to keep the pelvis parallel to the floor and (3) shaking.

2. The two functional exercises described in the text to strengthen hip abductors are sidestepping and side step-ups.

3. The advantage of testing the strength of hip adductors bilaterally in the frog-like supine position is that you can compare the left and right hips and therefore help determine what is normal hip strength for your client.

4. Whether performed in the standing or supine position, more strength is required to perform hip flexion with the knee extended.

5. Water-based exercises are helpful for someone with a hip problem because they can be used in the early stages of recovery to improve mobility and strength.

Chapter 8 Answers

1. Oedema, large thigh and calf muscles and fat deposits around the knee can all restrict active knee flexion.

2. When testing the strength of the knee extensors in either the sitting or prone position, gentle pressure can be applied to the anterior of the ankle to add resistance.

3. One advantage of performing an exercise to strengthen the knee extensors in the supine position with the hip flexed to approximately 90 degrees is that this helps to reduce swelling of the knee; one disadvantage is that it requires good flexibility in the hamstrings.

4. The stand-to-sit exercise is harder to perform than the sit-to-stand exercise because when we sit down, the quadriceps must work eccentrically, and this requires more effort than a concentric contraction (as in the sit-to-stand movement).

5. Once someone is able to perform a miniature squat against a wall, this could be progressed to a miniature squat without a wall, a deep squat with a wall, or a deep squat without a wall.

Chapter 9 Answers

1. Three advantages of a seated calf raise when treating someone with weak ankles or poor balance are that (1) it is manageable by most people, (2) it does not need to be performed bilaterally and (3) it does not require balance.

2. Heel walking strengthens the ankle dorsiflexor muscles.

3. It might be preferable to perform ankle evertor exercises bilaterally because this is easier than performing them unilaterally, irrespective of ankle strength.

4. Poor balance is indicated in the single-leg standing test when the duration for which a person can stand on their affected leg is reduced compared to the non-affected leg or when there is a lot of wobbling and the person must use their arms to maintain the position.

5. Examples of foot strengthening exercises used in foot gymnastics are using the feet and toes to tie a knot in a rope, using the toes to pick up and fasten a clothes peg to a line or to the edge of a cup, passing a stick or pencil back and forth with a partner, holding a paper cup between the toes of one foot whilst using the toes of the other foot to pick up small objects and deposit these in the cup or using the toes to pick up small hoops and place them over a pole.

Chapter 1

Adams, M.A., and W.C. Hutton. 1985. "The Effect of Posture on the Lumbar Spine." *Journal of Bone & Joint Surgery* 67 (4): 625-29.

American Academy of Orthopedic Surgeons. 2023. "Progressive Collapsed Foot Deformity (Flatfoot)." Accessed September 29, 2023. https://orthoinfo.aaos.org/en/diseases--conditions/posterior-tibial-tendon-dysfunction.

American College of Foot and Ankle Surgeons. 2023a. "Causes of Achilles Tendon Disorders." Accessed September 29, 2023. www.foothealthfacts.org/footankleinfo/achilles-tendon.htm.

American College of Foot and Ankle Surgeons. 2023b. "Cavus Foot (High-Arched Foot)." Accessed September 29, 2023. www.foothealthfacts.org/conditions/cavus-foot-(high-arched-foot).htm.

Betsch, M., J. Schneppendahl, L. Dor, P. Jungbluth, J.P. Grassmann, J. Windolf, S. Thelen, M. Hakimi, W. Rapp, and M. Wild. 2011. "Influence of Foot Positions on the Spine and Pelvis." *Arthritis Care & Research* 63 (12): 1758-65.

Beynnon, B.D., D.F. Murphy, and D.M. Alosa. 2002. "Predictive Factors for Lateral Ankle Sprains: A Literature Review." *Journal of Athletic Training* 37 (4): 376-380.

Bloomfield, J., T.R. Ackland, and B.C. Elliott. 1994. *Applied Anatomy and Biomechanics in Sport.* Victoria, Australia: Blackwell Scientific.

Burns, J., K.B. Landorf, M.M. Ryan, J. Crosbie, and R.A. Ouvrier. 2007. "Interventions for the Prevention and Treatment of Pes Cavus." *Cochrane Database of Systematic Reviews* 17 (14): CD006154. Accessed September 29, 2023. https://doi.org/10.1002/14651858.CD006154.pub2.

Cerejo, R., D.D. Dunlop, S. Cahue, D. Channin, J. Song, and L. Sharma. 2002. "The Influence of Alignment on Risk of Knee Osteoarthritis Progressing According to Baseline Stage of Disease." *Arthritis & Rheumatology* 46 (10): 2632-36.

Clementz, B.G. 1988. "Tibial Torsion Measured in Normal Adults." *Acta Orthopaedica Scandinavica* 59 (4): 441-42.

Cooperstein, R., and M. Lew. 2009. "The Relationship Between Pelvic Torsion and Anatomical Leg Length Discrepancy: A Review of the Literature." *Journal of Chiropractic Medicine* 8 (3): 107-13.

Corps, N., A.H. Robinson, R.L. Harrall, N.C. Avery, C.A. Curry, B.L. Hazleman, and G.P. Riley. 2012. "Changes in Matrix Protein Biochemistry and the Expression of mRNA Encoding Matrix Proteins and Metalloproteinases in Posterior Tibialis Tendinopathy." *Annals of the Rheumatic Diseases* 71 (5): 746-52.

Devan, M.R., L.S. Pescatello, P. Faghri, and J. Anderson. 2004. "A Prospective Study of Overuse Knee Injuries Among Female Athletes With Muscle Imbalances and Structural Abnormalities." *Journal of Athletic Training* 39 (3): 263-67.

Donatelli, R. 1987. "Abnormal Biomechanics of the Foot and Ankle." *Journal of Orthopaedic & Sports Physical Therapy* 9 (1): 11-16.

Fan, Y., Y. Fan, Z. Li, C. Lv, and D. Luo. 2011. "Natural Gaits of the Non-Pathological Flat Foot and High-Arched Foot." *PloS One* 6 (3): e17749. Accessed September 29, 2023. https://doi.org/10.1371/journal.pone.0017749.

Fish, D.J., and C.S. Kosta. 1998. "Genu Recurvatum: Identification of Three Distinct Mechanical Profiles." *Journal of Prosthetics and Orthotics* 10 (2): 26-32.

Fowler, R.P. 2004. "Recommendations for Management of Uncomplicated Back Pain in Workers' Compensation System: A Focus on Functional Restoration." *Journal of Chiropractic Medicine* 3 (4): 129-37.

Gandhi, S., R.K. Singla, J.S. Kullar, G. Agnihotri, V. Mehta, R.K. Suri, and G. Rath. 2014. "Human Tibial Torsion—Morphometric Assessment and Clinical Relevance." *Biomedical Journal* 37 (1): 10-13.

Giladi, M., C. Milgrom, M. Stein, H. Kashtan, J. Margulies, R. Chisin, R. Steinberg, R. Kedem, A. Aharonson, and A. Simkin. 1987. "External Rotation of the Hip: A Predictor of Risk for Stress Fractures." *Clinical Orthopaedics and Related Research* March (216): 131-34.

Gross, M.T. 1995. "Lower Quarter Screening for Skeletal Malalignment—Suggestions for Orthotics and Shoewear." *Journal of Orthopaedic & Sports Physical Therapy* 21 (6): 389-405.

Hagedorn, T.J., A.B. Dufour, J.L. Riskowski, H.J. Hillstrom, H.B. Menz, V.A. Casey, and M.T. Hannan. 2013. "Foot Disorder, Foot Posture and Foot Function: The Framingham Foot Study." *PLoS One* 8 (9): e74364. Accessed September 29, 2023. https://doi.org/10.1371/journal.pone.0074364.

Hicks, J., A. Arnold, F. Anderson, M. Schwartz, and S. Delp. 2007. "The Effect of Excessive Tibial Torsion on the Capacity of Muscles to Extend the Hip and Knee During Single-Limb Stance." *Gait & Posture* 26 (4): 546-52.

Houglum, P.A., and D.B. Bertoti. 2012. *Brunstromm's Clinical Kinesiology*. 6th ed. Philadelphia, PA: Davis.

Hughes, J., P. Clark, and L. Klenerman. 1990. "The Importance of Toes in Walking." *Journal of Bone & Joint Surgery British Volume* 72 (2): 245-51.

Inman, V.T. 1966. "Human Locomotion." *Canadian Medical Association Journal* 94 (4): 1047-54.

Jones, B.H., D.N. Cowan, J.P. Tomlinson, J.R. Robinson, D.W. Polly, and P.N. Frykman. 1993. "Epidemiology of Injuries Associated With Physical Training Among Young Men in the Army." *Medicine & Science in Sports & Exercise* 25 (2): 197-203.

Kapandji, A.I. 2008. *The Spinal Column, Pelvic Girdle and Head. The Physiology of the Joints*, vol. 3. London, UK: Churchill Livingstone.

Kendall, F.P., E.K. McCreary, and P.G. Provance. 1993. *Muscles: Testing and Function*. 4th ed. Baltimore, MD: Lippincott Williams and Wilkins.

Kerrigan, D.C., L.C. Deming, and M.K. Holden. 1996. "Knee Recurvatum in Gait: A Study of Associated Knee Biomechanics." *Archives of Physical Medicine and Rehabilitation* 77 (7): 645-50.

Levangie, P.K., and C.C. Norkin. 2001. *Joint Structure and Function: A Comprehensive Analysis*. Philadelphia, PA: Davis.

Levinger, P., H.B. Menz, M.R. Fotoohabadi, J.A. Feller, J.R. Bartlett, and N.R. Bergman. 2010. "Foot Posture in People With Medial Compartment Knee Osteoarthritis." *Journal of Foot and Ankle Research* 3 (29). Accessed September 29, 2023. https://doi.org/10.1186/1757-1146-3-29.

Levinger, P., H.B. Menz, A.D. Morrow, J.A. Feller, H.R. Bartlett, and N.R. Bergman. 2012. "Foot Kinematics in People With Medial Compartment Knee Osteoarthritis." *Rheumatology (Oxford)* 51 (12): 2191-98.

Loudon, J.K., H.L. Goist, and K.L. Loudon. 1998. "Genu Recurvatum Syndrome." *Journal of Orthopaedic & Sports Physical Therapy* 27 (5): 361-67.

Lun, V., W.H. Meeuwisse, P. Stergiou, and D. Stefanyshyn. 2004. "Relation Between Running Injury and Static Lower Limb Alignment in Recreational Runners." *British Journal of Sports Medicine* 38: 576-80.

Magee, D.J. 2002. *Orthopedic Physical Assessment*. 4th ed. Philadelphia, PA: Saunders.

McWilliams, D.F., S. Doherty, R.A. Maciewicz, K.R. Muir, W. Zhang, and M. Doherty. 2010. "Self-Reported Knee and Foot Alignments in Early Adult Life and Risk of Osteoarthritis." *Arthritis Care & Research* 62 (4): 489-95.

Mullaji, A.B., A.K. Sharma, S.V. Marawar, and A.F. Kohli. 2008. "Tibial Torsion in Non-Arthritic Indian Adults: A Computer Tomography Study of 100 Limbs." *Indian Journal of Orthopaedics* 42 (3): 309-13.

Myerson, M.S. 1996. "Adult Acquired Flatfoot Deformity: Treatment of Dysfunction of the Posterior Tibial Tendon." *Instructional Course Lectures* 46: 393-505.

Neumann, D.A. 2010. "Kinesiology of the Hip: A Focus on Muscular Actions." *Journal of Orthopaedic & Sports Physical Therapy* 40 (2): 82-94.

Riegger-Krugh, C., and J.J. Keysor. 1996. "Skeletal Malalignments of the Lower Quarter: Correlated and Compensatory Motions and Postures." *Journal of Orthopaedic & Sports Physical Therapy* 23 (2): 164-70.

Ritchie, G.W., and H.A. Keim. 1964. "A Radiographic Analysis of Major Foot Deformities." *Canadian Medical Association Journal* 91 (16): 840-44.

Samaei, A., A.H. Bakhtiary, F. Elham, and A. Rezasoltani. 2012. "Effects of Genu Varum Deformity on Postural Stability." *International Journal of Sports Medicine* 33 (6): 469-93.

Scannell, J.P., and S.M. McGill. 2003. "Lumbar Posture—Should It, and Can It, Be Modified? A Study of Passive Tissue Stiffness and Lumbar Position During Activities of Daily Living." *Physical Therapy* 83 (10): 907-17.

Sorensen, K.L., M.A. Holland, and E. Patla. 2002. "The Effects of Human Ankle Muscle Vibration on Posture and Balance During Adaptive Locomotion." *Experimental Brain Research* 143 (1): 24-34.

Strecker, W., P. Keppler, F. Gebhard, and L. Kinzl. 1997. "Length and Torsion of the Lower Limb." *Journal of Bone and Joint Surgery British Volume* 79 (6): 1019-23.

Tinkle, B.T. 2008. *Issues and Management in Joint Hypermobility*. Niles, IL: Left Paw Press.

Turner, M.S., and I.S. Smillie. 1981. "The Effect of Tibial Torsion on the Pathology of the Knee." *Journal of Bone and Joint Surgery British Volume* 63-B (3): 396-98.

Whitman, R. 2010. "The Classic: A Study of Weak Foot, With Reference to Its Causes, Its Diagnosis, and Its Cure, With an Analysis of a Thousand Cases of So-Called Flat-Foot 1896." *Clin Orthopedics and Related Research* 468 (4): 925-39.

Williams, D.S., I.S. McClay, and J. Hamill. 2001. "Arch Structure and Injury Patterns in Runners." *Clinical Biomechanics (Bristol, Avon)* 16 (4): 341-7.

Chapter 2

Binkley, J.M., P.W. Stratford, S.A. Lott, and D.L. Riddle. 1999. "The Lower Extremity Functional Scale (LEFS): Scale Development, Measurement Properties, and Clinical Application." *Physical Therapy* 79: 371-383.

Domsic, R.T., and C.L. Saltzman. 1998. "Ankle Osteoarthritis Scale." *Foot & Ankle International* 19 (7): 466-471.

Faculty of Pain Medicine and the British Pain Society. 2019. "Outcome Measures." January 2019. www.britishpainsociety.org/static/uploads/resources/files/Outcome_Measures_January_2019. pdf.

Greene, W.B., and J.D. Heckman. 1994. *The Clinical Measurement of Joint Motion*. Rosemont, IL: American Academy of Orthopaedic Surgeons.

Huguenin, L., P.D. Brukner, P. McCrory, P. Smith, H. Wajswelner, and K. Bennell. 2005. "Effect of Dry Needling of Gluteal Muscles on Straight Leg Raise: A Randomised, Placebo Controlled, Double Blind Trial." *British Journal of Sports Medicine* 39 (2): 84-90.

Irrgang, J.J., A.F. Anderson, A.L. Boland, C.D. Harner, M. Kurosaka, P. Neyret, J.C. Richmond, and K.D. Shelborne. 2001. "Development and Validation of the International Knee Documentation Committee Subjective Knee Form." *The American Journal of Sports Medicine* 29 (5): 600-13.

Kendall, F.P., E.K. McCreary, and P.G. Provance. 1993. *Muscles: Testing and Function*. 4th ed. Baltimore, MD: Lippincott Williams and Wilkins.

Madsen, L.P., E.A. Hall, and C.L. Docherty. 2018. "Assessing Outcomes in People With Chronic Ankle Instability: The Ability of Functional Performance Tests to Measure Deficits in Physical Function and Perceived Instability." *Journal of Orthopaedic & Sports Physical Therapy* 48 (5): 372-80.

Malliaropoulos, N., V. Korakakis, D. Christodoulou, N. Padhiar, D. Pyne, G. Giakas, T. Nauck, P. Malliaras, and H. Lohrer. 2014. "Development and Validation of a Questionnaire (FASH—Functional Assessment Scale for Acute Hamstring Injuries): To Measure the Severity and Impact of Symptoms on Function and Sports Ability in Patients With Acute Hamstring Injuries." *British Journal of Sports Medicine* 48 (22): 1607-12.

Martin, R.L., M.T. Cibulka, L.A. Bolgla, T.A. Koc Jr, J.K. Loudon, R.C. Manske, L. Weiss, J.J. Christoforetti, B.C. Heiderscheit, M. Voight, and J. DeWitt. 2022. "Hamstring Strain Injury in Athletes: Clinical Practice Guidelines Linked to the International Classification of Functioning, Disability and Health From the Academy of Orthopaedic Physical Therapy and the American Academy of Sports Physical Therapy of the American Physical Therapy Association." *Journal of Orthopaedic & Sports Physical Therapy* 52 (3): CPG1-44.

Mehta, S.P., A. Fulton, C. Quach, M. Thistle, C. Toledo, and N.A. Evans. 2016. "Measurement Properties of the Lower Extremity Functional Scale: A Systematic Review." *Journal of Orthopaedic & Sports Physical Therapy* 46 (3): 200-216.

Roos, E.M., and L.S. Lohmander. 2003. "The Knee Injury and Osteoarthritis Outcome Score (KOOS): From Joint Injury to Osteoarthritis." *Health and Quality of Life Outcomes* 1 (1): 1-8.

Scuderi, G.R., R.B. Bourne, P.C. Noble, J.B. Benjamin, J.H. Lonner, and W. Scott. 2012. "The New Knee Society Knee Scoring System." *Clinical Orthopaedics and Related Research* 470 (1): 3-19.

van de Hoef, P.A., M.S. Brink, N. van der Horst, M. van Smeden, and F.J.G. Backx. 2021. "The Prognostic Value of the Hamstring Outcome Score to Predict the Risk of Hamstring Injuries." *Journal of Science and Medicine in Sport* 24 (7): 641-6.

Willis, B., A. Lopez, A. Perez, L. Sheridan, and S. Kalish. 2009. "Pain Scale for Plantar Fasciitis." *The Foot and Ankle Online Journal* 2 (5): 3.

Chapter 3

Calvillo, A., G. Escalante, and M.J. Kolber. 2021. "The Relationship Between Hip Extensor Strength and Contralateral and Ipsilateral Hip Flexor Muscle Length in Healthy Men and Women." *The Sport Journal* 24: 1-10.

Ferguson, L. 2014. "Adult Idiopathic Scoliosis: The Tethered Spine." *Journal of Bodywork and Movement Therapies* 18: 99-111.

Gabbe, B.J., K.L. Bennell, and C.F. Finch. 2006. "Why Are Older Australian Football Players at Greater Risk of Hamstring Injury?" *Journal of Science and Medicine in Sport* 9 (4): 327-33.

Gulledge, B.M., D.J. Marcellin-Little, D. Levine, L. Tillman, O.L. Harrysson, J.A. Osborne, and B. Baxter. 2014. "Comparison of Two Stretching Methods and Optimization of Stretching Protocol for the Piriformis Muscle." *Medical Engineering & Physics* 36 (2): 212-18.

Oh, S., M. Kim, M. Lee, D. Lee, T. Kim, and B. Yoon. 2016. "Self-Management of Myofascial Trigger Point Release by Using an Inflatable Ball Among Elderly Patients With Chronic Low Back Pain: A Case Series." *Annals of Yoga and Physical Therapy* 1 (3): 1013.

Onik, G., T. Kasprzyk, K. Knapik, K. Wieczorek, D. Sieroń, A. Sieroń, A. Cholewka, and K. Sieroń. 2020. "Myofascial Trigger Points Therapy Modifies Thermal Map of Gluteal Region." *BioMed Research International* 2020: 4328253.

Chapter 4

Anandhi, D., T. Ansari, and V.P.R. Sivakumar. 2019. "Effectiveness of Tendoachilles and Hamstring Stretching on Nocturnal Leg Cramps Among Antenatal Women." *Global Journal of Physiotherapy and Rehabilitation* 1 (1): 1-8.

Espí-López, G., P. Serra-Año, J. Vicent-Ferrando, M. Sánchez-Moreno-Giner, J. Arias-Buria, J. Cleland, and C. Fernández-de-las-Peñas. 2017. "Effectiveness of Inclusion of Dry Needling in a Multimodal Therapy Program for Patellofemoral Pain: A Randomized Parallel-Group Trial." *Journal of Orthopaedic and Sport and Physical Therapy* 47 (6): 392-401.

Green, B., M.N. Bourne, N. van Dyk, and T. Pizzari. 2020. "Recalibrating the Risk of Hamstring Strain Injury (HSI): A 2020 Systematic Review and Meta-Analysis of Risk Factors for Index and Recurrent Hamstring Strain Injury in Sport." *British Journal of Sports Medicine* 54 (18): 1081-88.

Konrad, A., M. Nakamura, M. Tilp, O. Donti, and D.G. Behm. 2022. "Foam Rolling Training Effects on Range of Motion: A Systematic Review and Meta-Analysis." *Sports Medicine* 52 (10): 2523-35.

Prior, M., M. Guerin, and K. Grimmer. 2009. "An Evidence-Based Approach to Hamstring Strain Injury: A Systematic Review of the Literature." *Sports Health* 1 (2): 154-64.

Swash, M., D. Czesnik, and M. de Carvalho. 2019. "Muscular Cramp: Causes and Management." *European Journal of Neurology* 26 (2): 214-21.

Trampas, A., A. Kitsios, E. Sykaras, S. Symeonidis, and L. Lararous. 2010. "Clinical Massage and Modified Proprioceptive Neuromuscular Facilitation Stretching in Males With Latent Trigger Points." *Physical Therapy in Sport* 11 (3): 91-98.

Vachhani, R., and H. Sharma. 2021. "Effectiveness of Suboccipital Muscle Inhibition Technique Versus Muscle Energy Technique on Hamstring Muscle Flexibility in College Going Students." *International Journal of Research and Review* 8 (6): 160-74.

Chapter 5

Abdelmowla, R.A.A., H.A.A. Abdelmowla, and E.M. Fahem. 2022. "Iliotibial Band Friction Syndrome: Effect of Home Exercises on Patients' Clinical and Functional Outcomes." *Egyptian Journal of Health Care* 13 (2): 992-1001.

Anandhi, D., T. Ansari, and V.P.R. Sivakumar. 2019. "Effectiveness of Tendoachilles and Hamstring Stretching on Nocturnal Leg Cramps Among Antenatal Women." *Global Journal of Physiotherapy and Rehabilitation* 1 (1): 1-8.

Bannuru, R.R., M.C. Osani, E.E. Vaysbrot, N.K. Arden, K. Bennell, S.M.A. Bierma-Zeinstra, V.B. Kraus, et al. 2019. "OARSI Guidelines for the Non-Surgical Management of Knee, Hip, and Polyarticular Osteoarthritis." *Osteoarthritis and Cartilage* 27 (11): 1578-89.

Bloomfield, J., T.R. Ackland, and B.C. Elliott. 1994. *Applied Anatomy and Biomechanics of Sport.* Victoria, Australia: Blackwell Scientific.

Grieve, R., S. Barnett, N. Coghill, and F. Cramp. 2013. "Myofascial Trigger Point Therapy for Triceps Surae Dysfunction: A Case Series." *Manual Therapy* 18 (6): 519-25.

Grieve, R., A. Cranston, A. Henderson, G. Malone, and C. Mayall. 2013. "The Immediate Effect of Triceps Surae Myofascial Trigger Point Therapy on Restricted Active Ankle Joint Dorsiflexion in Recreational Runners: A Crossover Randomized Controlled Trial." *Journal of Bodywork Movement Therapies* 17: 453-61.

Gross, M.T. 1995. "Lower Quarter Screening for Skeletal Malalignment—Suggestions for Orthotics and Shoewear." *Journal of Orthopaedic & Sports Physical Therapy* 21 (6): 389-405.

Hutchinson, L.A., G.A. Lichtwark, R.W. Willy, and L.A. Kelly. 2022. "The Iliotibial Band: A Complex Structure With Versatile Functions." *Sports Medicine* 52 (5): 995-1008.

Kendall, F.P., E.K. McCreary, and P.G. Provance. 1993. *Muscles: Testing and Function.* 4th ed. Baltimore, MD: Lippincott Williams and Wilkins.

Kerrigan, D.C., L.C. Deming, and M.K. Holden. 1996. "Knee Recurvatum in Gait: A Study of Associated Knee Biomechanics." *Archives of Physical Medicine and Rehabilitation* 77 (7): 645-50.

Knight, I. 2011. *A Guide to Living With Hypermobility Syndrome.* Philadelphia, PA: Singing Dragon.

Kondrup, F., N. Gaudreault, and G. Venne. 2022. "The Deep Fascia and Its Role in Chronic Pain and Pathological Conditions: A Review." *Clinical Anatomy* 35 (5): 649-59.

Langendoen, J., and K. Sertel. 2011. *Kinesiology Taping*. Ontario, Canada: Robert Rose.

Lim, W.B., and O. Al-Dadah. 2022. "Conservative Treatment of Knee Osteoarthritis: A Review of the Literature." *World Journal of Orthopedics* 13 (3): 212.

Lin, X., F. Li, H. Lu, M. Zhu, and T.Z. Peng. 2022. "Acupuncturing of Myofascial Pain Trigger Points for the Treatment of Knee Osteoarthritis: A Systematic Review and Meta-Analysis." *Medicine* 101 (8): E28838.

Meek, W.M., M.P. Kucharik, C.T. Eberlin, S.A. Naessig, S.S. Rudisill, and S.D. Martin. 2022. "Calf Strain in Athletes." *JBJS Reviews* 10 (3): e21.

National Institute for Health and Clinical Excellence. 2022. "Osteoarthritis in Over 16s: Diagnosis and Management." NICE Guideline NG226. Accessed October 9, 2023. www.nice.org.uk/guidance/ng226.

Pavkovich, R. 2015. "The Use of Dry Needling for a Subject With Chronic Lateral Hip and Thigh Pain: A Case Report." *International Journal of Sports Physical Therapy* 10 (2): 246-55.

Rodrigues, P.T., A.F. Ferreira, R.M. Pereira, E. Bonfá, E.F. Borba, and R. Fuller. 2008. "Effectiveness of Medial-Wedge Insole Treatment for Valgus Knee Osteoarthritis." *Arthritis & Rheumatology* 15 (59): 603-8.

Rossi, A., S. Blaustein, J. Brown, K. Dieffenderfer, E. Ervine, S. Griffine, E. Firierson, K. Geist, and M. Johanson. 2017. "Spinal Peripheral Dry Needling Versus Peripheral Dry Needling Alone Among Individuals With a History of Ankle Sprain: A Randomized Controlled Trial." *International Journal of Sports Physical Therapy* 12 (7): 1034-47.

Shams Abrigh, H., and A. Moghaddami. 2020. "The Corrective Effect of an NASM Based Resistance Exercise on Genu Varum Deformity in Teenage Football Players." *DYSONA-Life Science* 1 (1): 14-19.

Swash, M., D. Czesnik, and M. de Carvalho. 2019. "Muscular Cramp: Causes and Management." *European Journal of Neurology* 26 (2): 214-21.

Watcharakhueankhan, P., G.J. Chapman, K. Sinsurin, T. Jaysrichai, and J. Richards. 2022. "The Immediate Effects of Kinesio Taping on Running Biomechanics, Muscle Activity, and Perceived Changes in Comfort, Stability and Running Performance in Healthy Runners, and the Implications to the Management of Iliotibial Band Syndrome." *Gait & Posture* 91: 179-85.

Wilke, J., L. Vogt, and W. Banzer. 2018. "Immediate Effects of Self-Myofascial Release on Latent Trigger Point Sensitivity: A Randomized, Placebo-Controlled Trial." *Biology of Sport* 35 (4): 349.

Chapter 6

Altomare, D., G. Fusco, E. Bertolino, R. Ranieri, C. Sconza, M. Lipina, E. Kon, et al. 2022. "Evidence-Based Treatment Choices for Acute Lateral Ankle Sprain: A Comprehensive Systematic Review." *European Review for Medical and Pharmacological Sciences* 26 (6): 1876-84.

American College of Foot and Ankle Surgeons. 2023a. "Flexible Flatfoot." Accessed October 16, 2023. www.foothealthfacts.org/conditions/flexible-flatfoot.

American College of Foot and Ankle Surgeons. 2023b. "Cavus Foot (High-Arched Foot)." Accessed October 16, 2023. www.foothealthfacts.org/conditions/cavus-foot-(high-arched-foot).

Arif, A., M.F. Afzal, T. Shahzadi, F. Nawaz, and I. Amjad. 2018. "Effects of Myofascial Trigger Point Release in Plantar Fasciitis for Pain Management." *Journal of Medical Sciences* 26 (2): 128-31.

Banwell, H.A., S. Mackintosh, and D. Thewlis. 2014. "Foot Orthoses for Adults With Flexible Pes Planus: A Systematic Review." *Journal of Foot and Ankle Research* 7 (1): 23. https://doi.org/10.1186/1757-1146-7-23.

Burns, J., K.B. Landorf, M.M. Ryan, J. Crosbie, and R.A. Ouvrier. 2007. "Interventions for the Prevention and Treatment of Pes Cavus." *Cochrane Database of Systematic Reviews* 2007 (4): CD006154. https://doi.org/10.1002/14651858.CD006154.pub2.

Donatelli, R. 1987. "Abnormal Biomechanics of the Foot and Ankle." *Journal of Orthopaedic Sports & Physical Therapy* 9 (1): 11-16.

Hartmann, A., K. Murer, R.A. de Bie, and E.D. de Bruin. 2009. "The Effect of a Foot Gymnastic Exercise Programme on Gait Performance in Older Adults: A Randomised Controlled Trial." *Disability and Rehabilitation* 31 (25): 2101-10. https://doi.org/10.3109/09638280902927010.

Jansen, H., M. Jordan, S. Frey, S. Hölscher-Doht, R. Meffert, and T. Heintel. 2018. "Active Controlled Motion in Early Rehabilitation Improves Outcome After Ankle Fractures: A Randomized Controlled Trial." *Clinical Rehabilitation* 32 (3): 312-18.

Kohls-Gatzoulis, J., J.C. Angel, D. Singh, F. Haddad, J. Livingstone, and G. Berry. 2004. "Tibialis Posterior Dysfunction: A Common Treatable Cause of Adult Acquired Flatfoot." *BMJ* 329 (7478): 1328-33.

Levangie, P.K., and C.C Norkin. 2001. *Joint Structure and Function: A Comprehensive Analysis.* Philadelphia, PA: Davis.

Luque-Suarez, A., G. Gijon-Nogueron, F.J. Baron-Lopez, M.T. Labajos-Manzanares, J. Hush, and M.J. Hancock. 2014. "Effects of Kinesiotaping in Foot Posture in Participants With Pronated Foot: A Quasi-Randomised Double-Blind Study." *Physiotherapy* 100 (1): 36-40.

Malvankar, S., W. Khan, A. Mahapatra, and G.S.E. Dowd. 2012. "How Effective Are Lateral Wedge Orthotics in Treating Medial Compartment Osteoarthritis of the Knee? A Systematic Review of Recent Literature." *Open Orthotics Journal* 6 (Suppl 3: M8): 544-47. https://doi.org/10.2174/1874325001206010544.

Manoli, A., and B. Graham. 2005. "The Subtle Cavus Foot, the 'Underpronator': A Review." *Foot & Ankle International* 26 (3): 256-63.

National Institute for Health and Clinical Excellence. 2020. "Sprains and Strains. Scenario: Management." Accessed October 11, 2023. https://cks.nice.org.uk/topics/sprains-strains/management/management.

Schneider, H.P., J.M. Baca, B.B. Carpenter, P.D. Dayton, A.E. Fleischer, and B.D. Sachs. 2018. "American College of Foot and Ankle Surgeons Clinical Consensus Statement: Diagnosis and Treatment of Adult Acquired Infracalcaneal Heel Pain." *The Journal of Foot and Ankle Surgery* 57 (2): 370-81.

Thummar, R.C., S. Rajaseker, and R. Anumasa. 2020. "Association Between Trigger Points in Hamstring, Posterior Leg, Foot Muscles and Plantar Fasciopathy: A Cross-Sectional Study." *Journal of Bodywork and Movement Therapies* 24 (4): 373-78.

Vicenzino, B., M. Franettovich, T. McPoil, T. Russell, G. Skardoon, and S. Bartold. 2005. "Initial Effects of Antipronation Tape on the Medial Longitudinal Arch During Walking and Running." *British Journal of Sports Medicine* 39 (12): 939-43.

Vuurberg, G., A. Hoorntje, L.M. Wink, B.F. Van Der Doelen, M.P. Van Den Bekerom, R. Dekker, C.D. Van Dijk, et al. 2018. "Diagnosis, Treatment and Prevention of Ankle Sprains: Update of an Evidence-Based Clinical Guideline." *British Journal of Sports Medicine* 52 (15): 956.

Wikstrom, E.A., M.S. Cain, A. Chandran, K. Song, T. Regan, K. Migel, and Z.Y. Kerr. 2021. "Lateral Ankle Sprain and Subsequent Ankle Sprain Risk: A Systematic Review." *Journal of Athletic Training* 56 (6): 578-85.

Chapter 9

Wagemans, J., C. Bleakley, J. Taeymans, A.P. Schurz, K. Kuppens, H. Baur, and D. Vissers. 2022. "Exercise-Based Rehabilitation Reduces Reinjury Following Acute Lateral Ankle Sprain: A Systematic Review Update With Meta-Analysis." *PloS One* 17 (2): e0262023.

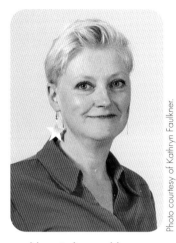

Photo courtesy of Kathryn Faulkner.

Jane Johnson, PhD, MSc, BSc(Hons), BA(Hons), CSP, HCPC, is a chartered physiotherapist specializing in occupational health and massage. In this role she assesses the posture of clients; performs manual assessments, including that of the soft tissues; and determines whether work, sport, or recreational postures may be contributing to a person's symptoms. She devises postural correction plans that include both hands-on and hands-off techniques. A key element of her work involves educating each client in how to self-manage their condition.

Johnson has taught continuing professional development workshops for organizations in the United Kingdom and abroad. This experience has brought her into contact with thousands of therapists of varying disciplines and has informed her own practice. Johnson has a particular passion for inspiring and supporting students and newly qualified therapists to gain confidence in the use of assessment and treatment techniques.

Johnson is a member of the Chartered Society of Physiotherapy and is registered with the Health and Care Professions Council. For many years she provided expert witness reports on cases involving soft tissue therapies. Johnson is the author of six titles in the Hands-On Guides for Therapists series: *Postural Assessment*, *Postural Correction*, *Therapeutic Stretching*, *Soft Tissue Release*, *Deep Tissue Massage* and *Soft Tissue and Trigger Point Release*. These titles have been translated into multiple different languages, including Japanese, traditional Chinese, simplified Chinese, Korean, German, Italian, Spanish and Portuguese. *Postural Assessment* has sold over 15,000 copies. Johnson is also the author of *The Big Back Book: Tips & Tricks for Therapists*.

Johnson regularly delivers webinars on popular musculoskeletal topics as well as on life working as a therapist. In her Facebook group, 'Jane Johnson: The Friendly Physio', she shares tips and tricks in her usual friendly manner.

Johnson lives in the north of England in an unmodernized house, where she creates books and webinars, keeps a sketchbook and nature journal, and rehomes big rescue dogs. Her Instagram page is @janejohnson5047, 'The physio who keeps a sketchbook'.

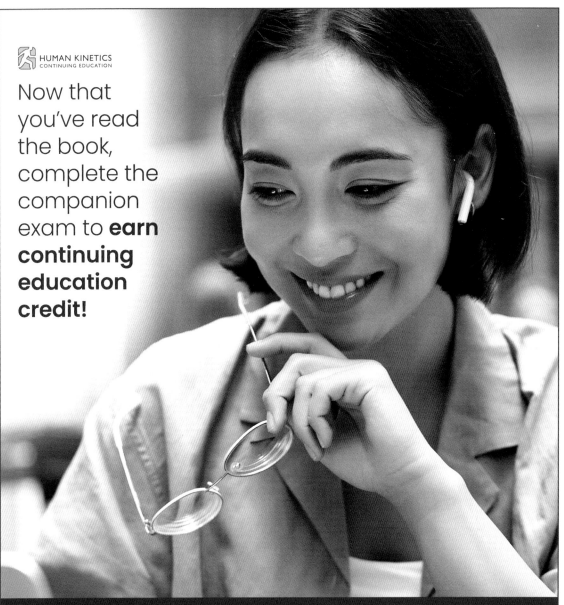
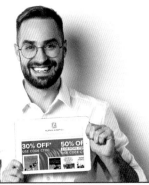